Dear Marie,

Compl...
Diss...
Co...

LIVING WELL WITH CHRONIC ILLNESS

Jan. 2001

Romans 12:12

Sincerely in Christ,

Marcia

Practical help and Resources for . . .

LIVING
WELL
WITH
CHRONIC
ILLNESS

Marcia Van't Land

Harold Shaw Publishers
Wheaton, Illinois

ISBN 0-87788-761-6

Cover design and illustration Copyright © 1994 by David LaPlaca

Library of Congress Cataloging-in-Publication Data

Van't Land, Marcia.
Living well with chronic illness / Marcia Van't Land.
    p. cm.
   Includes bibliographical references.
   ISBN 0-87788-761-6
   1. Chronic diseases—Popular works. 2. Chronically ill. 3. Chronic diseases—Religious aspects—Christianity. I. Title.
   RC108.V37 1994
   362.1'96—dc20

           93—10903
           CIP

99 98 97 96 95 94

10 9 8 7 6 5 4 3 2 1

*This project is dedicated
to everyone who has helped
me on my journey.*

Contents

Part One

Coming to Terms with Chronic Illness

1

The Chronic Condition

*When you pass through the waters, I will be
with you; and when you pass through the
rivers, they will not sweep over you.—Isaiah
43:2*

In early 1980, I was a healthy thirty-two-year-old wife and
mother of three preschool children. I spent a week in the
hospital during a severe case of the flu. Afterward I went on
with my busy family life and we made a cross-country move.
I blamed my fatigue and back pain on the fact that I was busy
with moving and didn't get enough rest. Soon my feet began
to flop when I walked. I'd be holding our baby and have to set
her down before I dropped her. Finally, I went to a neurologist
and he immediately put me in the hospital. My body stopped
functioning and they attached me to a respirator with the
diagnosis of Guillian Barre' Syndrome, a debilitating neurological disease of the central nervous system caused by a
virus. They surmised that my body had harbored the flu virus
and it had traveled into my nervous system.

Over the next two months I recovered somewhat. But the
fatigue and pain finally sent me back to the neurologist. He
could feel the muscle spasms in my back and legs, so he gave
me three injections of cortisone. While he was giving me the
third injection, I passed out and had several seizures.

I went into the hospital doubled over with abdominal
pain. My bladder and bowels stopped working. They

performed every test in the book and the doctors suspected I had recurring Guillian Barre' Syndrome. I came home from a three-week hospital stay pained and confused. About ten days later my neurologist called to inform me that my three delta ALA tests showed a hundred times above the normal reading. This was an indication of a rare disease called porphyria. He consulted another doctor who knew more about porphyria.

We learned that acute intermittent porphyria was one of seven porphyrias. Possible symptoms of the disease: severe abdominal pain, nausea, vomiting, constipation, pain in the back, legs, and arms, muscle weakness (due to the effects on nerves supplying the muscles), urinary retention, palpitation due to rapid heartbeat often accompanied by increased blood pressure, confusion, hallucinations, and seizures (myoclonus in my case).

There is no cure for AIP, but if one stays away from certain drugs, the disease can go into remission. Hospitalization is often necessary for acute attacks. Medication is needed for pain, nausea, and vomiting. Close observation is generally required because of respiratory distress. A high intake of glucose, other carbohydrates, or hematin—given intravenously—can help suppress disease activity.

Due to all the attacks I've experienced, I have been hospitalized more than forty times over a period of eleven years. I have been in the ICU many times. I have severe neuromuscular damage and need a wheelchair. Often my breathing is affected, necessitating that I have oxygen at home. I've had numerous surgeries, one of which resulted in the removal of my badly diseased bladder.

My skin is very sensitive and I often have lesions, called pernio, on my chest, neck, face, arms, and toes.

My auto-immune system is suppressed and I have frequent infections throughout my body. Various organs such as my kidneys do not function well.

We have consulted doctors at four medical centers, but the answer is always the same: "Mrs. Van't Land, we can't do anything but treat the symptoms as they occur."

At first my doctor said that I only had two or three years to live. Then he said five. Now he doesn't predict a time frame. He calls me his challenge and a "miracle woman." Each day I thank God for my miracle.

What Is a Chronic Condition?

Webster defines *chronic* as "marked by long duration of frequent recurrence: always present." Because of our advances in medical care, people are living longer and are surviving illnesses that were once immediate killers. The longer a person lives, the more apt he or she is to develop a chronic illness or disability.

For the purposes of this book "chronic condition" means:

- permanent
- the cause of frequent and costly medical intervention
- the cause of substantial modification of lifestyle, life goals, vocational choices and opportunities, recreational activities, interpersonal relationships, family role or position[1]

There are more than thirty-five million disabled people in our country. In 1980, in the U.S. alone, seventy-five million Americans had back problems. Each year seven million people are added to this list. Of these, five million are partially disabled and two million are unable to work. In addition to these statistics more than sixty million Americans deal daily with chronic illness. It is impossible to include a comprehensive list of all illnesses and disabilities that fit into those categories:

- Lupus and its various forms
- Emphysema
- Cancer
- Diabetes
- Heart disease
- Parkinson's
- Cystic fibrosis
- Alzheimer's
- AIDS
- Multiple sclerosis
- Stroke with permanent damage
- Severe asthma
- Back problems
- Arthritis
- Epilepsy
- Orphan diseases
- Spina bifida
- Dystrophies severe enough to impair
- Neurological diseases (Lou Gehrig's, Guillain Barre' Syndrome)
- Mental illness (not included in the sixty million listed above)
- Prolonged coma from any number of causes
- Eating disorders

Treatments for cancer have advanced so rapidly that this disease is now classified as a chronic illness; once in remission, it can lie dormant for months or even years before reappearing.

In her book, *It's Always Something,* Gilda Radner says, "Fighting cancer is a continuing process like controlling diabetes or any other chronic disease. I have to continue to fight it. I can't ever stop. I can't ever let down and say, 'I beat it. I licked it. I'm finished.'"[2]

Chronic situations can produce many new stresses and challenges to a person and his family and friends. People with a chronic illness or disability go through the phases of grief many, many times. It is an up-and-down world that never goes away.

Part of my frustration is the scarcity of information available to me. My disease is an *orphan disease,* meaning that it affects less than 200,000 people in the United States. There are more than 5,000 debilitating orphan diseases that afflict approximately twenty million Americans today.

The Birth of a Book

Recently I went to a large public library and counted hundreds of books in their medical section. Although there were books on the many specific diseases, there were none on chronic situations in general and how to cope with them. Of the five books on my research list, not even one was on the shelf. There just isn't much material available for those whose medical problems are long-term and/or recurring.

How can we go on year after year? How do we cope with nonstop medical bills? How do we handle the fact that my symptoms will increase rather than improve? *What are we supposed to do?*

We must learn to live with the circumstances, do the best we can, and make adjustments. Gathering information about our situations often enlightens us to make more intelligent decisions. From time to time we must evaluate our decisions and make some changes.

It was out of this mindset that this book was born. The pregnancy lasted eleven very difficult years, and the labor pains were intense. But I have tried to produce a book especially for people in chronic situations—we'll call them "situationers."

In the time that we (reader and author) will spend together, we'll fluctuate through the ups and downs of living with a chronic situation. Where can we turn when we, or a loved one, becomes a chronic situationer?

We'll discover that our symptoms and inner thoughts are genuine, not figments of our imaginations. We'll learn how to live with rearranged bodies and in what ways we can still be useful in our family, community, and church life.

We will examine the role of the medical profession and how our health-care teams can provide assistance.

Important decisions for the chronic situationer and his family will be closely inspected. After this time together we can go on with our lives, without the blinders that make us focus on just ourselves.

With all the information we can collect, all the strategies we can conceive, and all the loving help we can receive from friends and family, ultimately we would never keep going if we didn't have a God who cared about each one of us. The state of our spiritual health is of utmost importance to our health in general. For this reason I quote Scripture unashamedly throughout this book; it has been my strength and continues to give comfort and wisdom. We depend on the mercy, grace, and help of God as we endeavor to live fruitfully—not merely survive—with chronic illness.

Encouragement along the Way

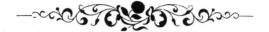

*"T*herefore, since we have a great high priest who has gone through the heavens, Jesus the Son of God, let us hold firmly to the faith we profess. For we do not have a high priest who is unable to sympathize with our weaknesses, but we have one who has been tempted in every way, just as we are—yet was without sin. Let us then approach the throne of grace with confidence, so that we may receive mercy and find grace to help us in our time of need."—Hebrews 4:14-16

2

What Is Wrong with Me?

Let him who walks in the dark, who has no light, trust in the name of the LORD and rely on his God.—Isaiah 50:10

Have an ongoing, incurable illness? No, not me. I was Marcia, the athlete, teacher, coach, wife, mother, and friend. I prided myself on being trim and in-shape. I visited the sick in hospitals and nursing homes. I sent cards and wrote encouraging letters to those who were involved in tragic circumstances.

Now I was a physical misfit. My feet flopped when I walked. I was no longer in control of my body.

Secretly I knew something was wrong with my central nervous system. I contracted shingles when our children had chicken pox, which is unusual for a healthy thirty-year-old. Shingles and chicken pox are caused by the same virus. I also knew that my week-long hospital stay for a case of the flu was unusual. I didn't breathe a word of these fears to anyone but God. He knew anyway.

My journal entry of April 1983:

As I lay in the Intensive Care Unit attached to a respirator—

Neurologist: "*I feel that Marcia has Guillian Barre' Syndrome. She didn't have any reflexes last night.*"

Internist: "*No, I don't think so. All the symptoms don't check out.*"

A few days later after the test results—

Neurologist: "*I'm not sure what happened. All her tests are clear and she's improving.*"

Internist: "*I feel that we are seeing a case of psychosomatic illness. She isn't really ill. I would like to call in a psychiatrist.*"

Neurologist: "*O.K. Go ahead and we'll see what happens.*"

Psychiatrist: "*Do you mind if I ask you a few questions?*"

Me: "*Sure, that's fine.*"

The internist wrote this diagnosis on my medical records:

"*Psychosomatic Illness Resembling Guillian Barre' Syndrome*"

From then on I was DOOMED wherever my medical records went. I spent many hours doubting myself. Like a good patient I tried to ignore my constant pain. I was exhausted but I would push myself to keep going. And when I couldn't, I'd push some more. I was trapped in a deteriorating body and the medical profession didn't believe me. I desperately needed someone to think I was still sane.

Usually when we go to a doctor he examines us and tells what he found and suggests treatment or more diagnostic procedures. Sometimes the doctor can't tell what is wrong. Medical science does have its limits and diagnosis can be difficult.

The doctor may recommend that we come to see him in a few days or weeks, if we don't feel better. He is saying that he doesn't think we are in any immediate danger and time will tell what is wrong.

The Mystery of Medical Diagnosis

Every person involved in a chronic situation has a different story to tell. Some have been diagnosed very quickly and didn't go through the medical rigamarole of going from doctor to doctor looking for an answer. Others of us have gone on for years without any answers. Our families and friends begin to believe that our symptoms are all in our heads.

Our symptoms can be vague and mimic other diseases. Some illnesses progress slowly like Parkinson's, lupus, or arthritis. Often a person partially recovers between attacks and test results come out within a normal range, meaning that a diagnosis cannot be made. My neurologist really persevered with us. He was caring and he believed me when I told him my symptoms; he did not want to label me with a disease before he had more information. He suspected something was wrong in my body and was as frustrated as we were. He did stress, however, that I learn to live with my undiagnosed illness until there was more evidence.

Being a medical mystery can be devastating. We get on a merry-go-round of specialists, tests, and treatments. A person with a rare disease or one that is difficult to diagnose needs to take control of his or her health and become a medical detective. When that is necessary there are some practical steps to keep in mind.

Being Your Own Medical Detective

1. Find a good general practitioner. It's best if you have a doctor familiar with you before you have symptoms. If the generalist can't solve your mystery, let him refer you to specialists. He should continue to guide the rest of your treatment; he sees you as a whole person, while specialists see only part of you.

2. Believe in yourself. You know better than anyone when something is wrong; don't back down if doctors suggest that it is psychosomatic. Not having others believe in us is one of the most difficult issues we deal with.

3. Keep a list of symptoms, tests, and treatments, including the day and time of each. Where were you when symptoms flared up? What were you doing? Medical diaries can reveal patterns that indicate allergies and asthma, occupational illness, and other conditions. Make sure this list also contains any old injuries and diseases you've had. Family medical history is also an important guide. List

any diseases that may run in your family. *Only take this list out when you have a doctor who will listen to you.* Otherwise you may be labeled a hypochondriac. Even if it serves no other purpose, this list will bring you some peace of mind.

4. Make a list of every drug you take and keep it with you. It provides valuable information for the doctor. Sometimes the dosages can be wrong or two drugs may fight each other within your body. Make sure you mention any over-the-counter medications, including vitamins and minerals.

5. Reevaluate your lifestyle and job conditions. Does anyone you work with have these same symptoms? Are you allergic to your pets? How much coffee do you drink? Have you been on an out-of-country trip? Maybe you're allergic to the dust caused by your house remodeling?

6. Read, read, read. Go to your local library and research diseases. Some doctors provide literature, but there are medical research services available that have more information.

Your librarian should be able to help you. Read health magazines and medical books. Often when a person is a medical mystery, he can diagnose himself and present this to the doctor. Some doctors don't appreciate this, so wait until you've established a working relationship with your doctor.

7. Are there stresses and emotional factors in your life that could be causing some of your symptoms? Stress alone can cause a number of physical symptoms, and if you think that might be happening, an appointment with a counselor is not out of line. I think we balk at seeing a psychiatrist because it implies there is no physical problem causing the symptoms. No one likes to be taken lightly and shipped off to some other doctor. Psychotherapy is helpful in many cases and does not suggest that we are crazy.[1] Psychological symptoms can sometimes be the missing link in correct diagnosis of the physical condition.

The Reality of Diagnosis

I could feel the lead weight in my stomach when, by exclusion of everything else, I knew I had porphyria. In my friend's nursing book there was only one highly technical paragraph.

When a diagnosis is finally made of a debilitating condition, we can at first be shocked and numb, but in most cases we've already suspected a serious disease before it had a name. Now it's really true and we must deal with it.

When we are in this situation we can become overwhelmed. We might be so confused that we forget to ask questions and so come home not remembering exactly what the doctor told us. We may need time to think, gather some information, and consider the options that are available. In most medical problems, a delay of a day or two won't affect the cause of the disorder. After some time to think you can call or make an appointment to discuss treatment.

> Sometimes it is hard to find the truth. What is harder is trying not to run away from it when we've found it.—Marcia Van't Land

On our good days we can pretend we don't have diabetes, heart disease, or some other debilitating condition. But gradually more symptoms occur and we know that we cannot ignore them. Some get their back against a wall and say, "I'll disobey my doctor's orders to stay in bed. I'm not going to take my medicine. I'll show everyone that I can beat this."

In *Total Care of Spinal Cord Injuries* the author says "that often their patients will say, 'I am not really paralyzed' or 'I will walk out of their hospital cured.' " [2] The patient involves himself in wishful thinking by denying that circumstances have changed his life. If we get stuck in this denial phase, we will never deal effectively with the chronic situation. We cannot make adjustments and go on with our lives. We are continually angry and frustrated.

Two years after my disease surfaced, I still denied that it existed. I had lesions on my skin and especially on my toes. It baffled my dermatologist and she sent me to a medical school clinic. About eight medical students came in, looked at my toes, asked me questions, and then wrote their diagnosis of the pernio condition. All of them asked, "Are you in good health?" Eight times I had to answer, "No, I have acute intermittent porphyria." I wanted to stagger out the door, stop all the traffic, and angrily yell, "I have porphyria! Do you hear me? I have porphyria!" Being forced into admitting that I had porphyria led me to accept that fact. That is when I stopped denying the truth.

> *We cannot change the diagnosis but we can choose the attitude with which we will deal with it.*
> *—Robert Cantor* [3]

When our good health disappears it rattles us. Everyone involved in a chronic situation grieves. We mourn the loss of walking, the use of our arms, of breathing on our own. We mourn the loss of our once active spouse or parent. It's extremely sad to know that the uncertainty of our health will always be with us until we get to heaven. It hurts so much.

Grieving for what we've lost is normal and nothing to be ashamed of. In my case I didn't have much time or space to grieve because of my busy, young family. As a result I kept a stiff upper lip. Several years into my illness, I finally realized I no longer had the energy to protect my family and friends from my disease. I stopped pretending and let them see my struggle. It shocked some friends and I never saw or heard from them again. Perhaps they felt guilty and didn't want to be reminded of their own mortality.

Grief is not something we recover from. It is a process and there are times when we feel like we've lost everything and everyone. However, we can come to see that losses in life are inevitable and we must cultivate understanding, compassion, and courage in the midst of our losses. We think we should be handling these losses better. We keep thinking, *What am I doing wrong?*

Don't I Have Enough Faith?

While sitting in my wheelchair one day, eating cake and ice cream at a fiftieth wedding anniversary party, a woman, whom I had never met, bent down and said, "Your faith isn't strong enough. If you had more faith you wouldn't need that wheelchair." I was so flabbergasted I couldn't respond as I watched her walk out the door.

Over the years I've had several people wanting to take me to a faith healer to see if he or she could heal me from my disease. I always responded, "No. I believe that if and when God wants to heal me, it will be among my own friends and relatives and in the church I attend." I've never felt this intense desire to go from church to church seeking healing.

Jim, whose love for the Lord shines in his eyes, has lived with debilitating arthritis for twenty-two years. Every movement pains him and he is very limited in a physical way, but he keeps a detailed prayer list and is a faithful prayer warrior.

Before her car accident, Karen used her God-given talents to compose, sing, and accompany others in Christian entertainment. Now she has lost the use of her legs, her singing voice, and has limited arm strength. She maintains a positive attitude and now writes and composes using a computer stick.

One of my friends has multiple sclerosis. She had a minister and elders pray and anoint her with oil as it says in James 5:14: "Is any one of you sick? He should call the elders of the church to pray over him and anoint him with oil in the name of the Lord." My friend was not healed of her MS, but she did feel a spiritual healing and was able to get beyond the question of "Why?" She felt more at peace within herself and with God.

Do my friends and I lack faith? Was my disease and the illness or accident of others a cruel joke on us because of some apparent sins?

There aren't personal reasons for every problem in life. God doesn't operate that way. Sometimes we suffer simply because we have frail, human bodies. To be human and live in a fallen world guarantees that we will suffer tragedies. It is true that our physical well-being is affected by our emotional and spiritual health; for instance, bitterness and anxiety often figure into stress-related diseases. But unless God reveals some specific wrongdoing on our part—or shows us a wrong pattern of living that has affected our health—it is not for us to draw connections between our medical problems and our standing with God. We can drive ourselves crazy trying to figure out why things happen as they do.

> *[I] believe that the healing miracles we pray for*
> *are performed in the attitudes, behaviors, and the*
> *life styles of the afflicted, i.e., how we handle the*

> *stress, discomforts, frustrations of a particular*
> *undesirable condition rather than the absence of*
> *pain, disease, injury, or so.—Dr. Lewis Smedes*[4]

Do I think we should believe in miracles? Of course. Our God is capable of performing a miracle at any time and place. God has the power to accomplish his purposes over a period of time or instantaneously. We do not know what God has in mind for us and he can and will use our circumstances. God cannot be limited by our human minds.

In the last eleven years I have seen some purpose to my suffering. One woman broke her ankle while she was out in the dairy pasture. No one was home and she had to crawl to the house. What kept her going was the chant, "If Marcia can do it, I can do it. If Marcia can do it, I can do it." Another friend thanked me for allowing her to honestly see my hurts and joys. She felt that watching our family over the years helped prepare their family when a long-term situation came to reside in their family.

I have no doubt that my faith could heal me. But I must trust that the condition I find my body in is one that God can use. My faith reminds me that God loves me so much that whatever situations I face, I can trust him, confident that he will never forsake me and will give his comfort to me. I have a deeper relationship with God now than I did when I was healthy. I must rely on God completely, and when I do he can accomplish his purposes in my life.

God sees the whole picture of which we are only a small part. He is the King of the universe, the all-knowing Sovereign, the Almighty. He has said that he loves us . . . and he sent his only Son to prove it. It is like Jesus checked into this great big hospital where we all live. He became a patient just like us. And the more we learn about the suffering Jesus went through, the more help he gives us for what we ourselves must endure.

It is always comforting to know that God grieves, too. Jesus grieved. In John 11:33-36 we read that he wept at the death of Lazarus. He wept when he looked over Jerusalem, knowing what was going to happen there.

Jesus is kind to those who are grieving. He doesn't say, "Now, get over it. Snap out of it." He says to the woman who was healed from a long-term illness by touching Jesus' garment, "Your faith has healed you. Go in peace and be freed from your suffering" (Mark 5:34).

I still mourn whenever I see families riding bikes together. I'm jealous. I want to teach our kids how to play tennis and volleyball, but I must be content to let others do that.

Sometimes I get angry when people gawk at me in my wheelchair. They're afraid to touch me or be close to me. But my anger is often unleashed at those I love the most— my family, friends, medical care personnel. I get tired of living with my rearranged body. The kids will ask, "Mom, what's wrong?" I reply, "ME!"

Sometimes in my anger I ask, "Has God forsaken me? Is my faith weak?" I doubt that I can bear this disease nobly. I'm reassured when I'm told that my questions are signs of a deepening faith—a struggle to believe that Christ is Lord and that he will provide what we need to grow beyond our tragedies, if we trust him.

After my anger subsides, I rest in the fact that through my adversity I am learning to know the touch of God and that in his eyes I'm his child—not some oddball creation.

> *It is not what we know (even the whys) but whom we know, that is critical to our survival.—Stanley C. Baldwin*[5]

I am thankful for being born into a Christian family. What I learned and established by regular study of God's Word provides me with valuable armor for the battle that will not end during this life. Jesus is with us on long, painful, dark nights. He speaks comforting words in Matthew 11:28: "Come to me, all you who are weary and burdened, and I will give you rest." For those of us in long-term situations that is the only rest we will find on this earth.

We can still have faith while we're hurting—a faith that focuses on God. A faith that leads to positive actions. A faith that brings us outside ourselves so that we can comfort a person with similar problems. A faith that knows that God loves us completely—right where we are.

Encouragement along the Way

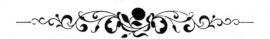

Scripture songs I've memorized over the years have often kept me going. Whenever I am lying in the hospital, weak and pained, my aunt will whisper to me, "I'll go home and play your favorite hymns on my organ." I can hear the organ in my mind:

He giveth more grace when the burdens grow greater.
He sendeth more strength when the labors increase;
To added affliction He addeth His mercy,
To multiplied trials, His multiplied peace.

When we have exhausted our store of endurance,
When our strength has failed ere the day is half done,
When we reach the end of our hoarded resources,
Our Father's full giving is only begun.

His love has no limit, His grace has no measure.
His power has no boundary known unto men;
For out of His infinite riches in Jesus.
He giveth, and giveth, and giveth again.
—Annie Johnson Flint[6]

3

This Is How I Feel

Everyone should be quick to listen, slow to speak.— James 1:19

The majority of people in the world grow up able-bodied. That means their physical being develops, strengthens, and performs as it was designed to do. While some people are grateful for this gift, most take it for granted or automatically assume they will be in good physical health."[1]

Many of us have years of living with a chronic situation under our belts. We have made all kinds of adjustments. We use whatever aids are necessary, we've learned to cope, and we've done the best we could with what we have.

We've also worked hard at being useful people. We have many valuable experiences from which others can learn. But they can only learn from us if they listen to us.

It's trite to say, but if you've never been ill, you don't notice—or enjoy—not being ill.—Claudia Black[2]

Chronically ill people are in a never-ending and confusing process. The changes we experience emotionally can be intimidating to the people around us. In the first months after diagnosis one feels like nothing will ever be the same again. In a sense we're right. Everything will now be seen through the cracked glasses of chronic illness or accident. It affects us physically, psychologically, spiritually, and financially. It is not just a history, some test results, and prescriptions that lie in a folder in the doctor's office. It affects our most important relationships and can turn our whole lives upside down. Will the ill person gradually take over the well part and alter our lives? Our chances of being as "well" as possible are much better when we can face the various emotions and voice them to those who would support us.

We Feel Fear

Fear is one of the most unpleasant emotions that we experience as part of a loss. The experience of the loss of our health can make us fear for our well-being or safety, and it creates uncertainty about the future; we're afraid that we will lose more.

Nearly everyone who is in a chronic situation experiences fear but won't admit it. My mind goes crazy and I imagine myself wasting away in a convalescent home, unable to care for myself. When we see others with our disease or a similar one and see the progression of their disease, it can make us afraid: *Is that going to happen to me?*

We can never say, "I'm cured," unless God sends a miracle. Even when all symptoms are gone and we're in a remission, we know that the disease will probably return in a different form. We fear the uncertainty, and planning ahead is almost impossible.

I am alarmed when I think how my body has changed over the last twelve years. I was always active and could eat what I wanted without gaining weight. Will my family still love me when my body has changed?

I am afraid of losing control. The hardest part of living with a chronic condition is carrying it around for years. It weighs heavy and sometimes I want to escape from it. No matter what I do, I can't seem to get out from under it.

Every time I end up in ICU again my fear intensifies with the knowledge that my time is running out. I realize I haven't done all I want to do. It is irritating to have to stay in bed when the sunshine invites me outside. What can be more frustrating than being cooped up or immobilized in a cast or traction?

> *Fear comes creeping up my bones and makes my bones go soft.—Unknown*

One of my hospital roommates asked me, "How can you keep going year after year?" I told her there is only one way to do it: just bear it. I bear it and go on because what else am I going to do? I don't have an alternative. But I am afraid for the future. Because of this stress some of us become nervous, have bad dreams, or sudden panic attacks. This is normal for someone in a chronic situation.

Facing our own death can be a frightening experience also. We are constantly reminded that our body is frail. Life is short and we have little control over what happens to us in this life.

Bernice Wallin, in her book *I Beat Cancer,* says, "Whenever I felt a pain somewhere in my body, my heart skipped a beat or two and I was afraid that the cancer had returned."[3] This is one of the ways that the fear of dying often expresses itself.

Often our ever-so-common fear of death leads us to put our fate in the hands of the doctor. "Please save me." Some go from doctor to doctor hoping for a better prognosis. But doctors need to remind us that they are human and have scientific limitations. Words echo in my mind: *I'm sorry Mrs. Van't Land. There is nothing we can do except treat the symptoms as they occur. We don't know how the disease will progress.*

We Feel Anger

As a result of fear we often become angry. Usually we're not angry at a certain person. We're mad at ourselves, our bodies, our situations, even at God. We often take our emotions out on the people closest to us—in the form of angry outbursts. Please remember that our anger is a normal reaction to limited activity and we don't want to hurt anyone.

I get angry and frustrated when I don't have the energy to be up and around at home. I become quiet and sullen. I show no enthusiasm for life and cannot bear to hear another story like mine. When I pull back in that way, I don't mean to be insensitive to others. I just cannot endure more shadows hanging over me.

I wish so much to have a normal functioning body, and that leaves me very little patience for those who knowingly abuse their bodies and minds. I always pray that I will still be able to show love for these people. But I also pray that at the same time I can impress upon them the message that life is precious and is not to be wasted.

Sometimes I feel cheated—that my body is failing me when I'm so young. I have filled many tear bottles that God is storing up for me in heaven (see Psalm 56:8, RSV). When I get to heaven God is going to give me the privilege and satisfaction of emptying these bottles over the cliff and smashing them to bits on the rocks below. Then my anger and fear will be totally gone.

We Feel Alone

When someone is diagnosed with a form of cancer or a rare terminal disease, you can see the terror in people's eyes. Just the thought of meeting someone in a wheelchair and not knowing how to act can make others want to remove themselves from your presence. Some are afraid to touch or comfort when the patient needs comforting the most. Many are "scared *to* death" of us because they themselves are scared *of* death. They don't want to be confronted with the idea that life is not fair and all people must die. And the best way to avoid these feelings is to physically avoid the person and his family. Chronically ill persons don't want to scare anyone. They want—just like others—to live as long as they can and make the most of their lives.

It is normal to lose acquaintances through the years of a chronic situation. (Notice I said, "acquaintances.") It's also normal for our friendships to change as we adjust to our altered lifestyle. Prolonged and repeated hospitalizations weed out all but the most committed visitors.

My husband, Tom, and I experienced isolation when we went through one medical clinic after another. No one really knew our pain and fears—our nightmares—except God. We mourned the loss of my health and how it affected our family. Tom had to deal with the fear and possibility of losing me—the only adult who truly knew him. We also experienced isolation as news of my illness spread. People didn't know what to say as I struggled from year to year, progressively getting worse. Distorted gossip had me dead and buried several times. We felt as if we lived in our own little nightmarish world with everyone looking in.

I wish there were windows to my soul, so that you could see some of my feelings.—Artimus Ward

Dr. Howard Vanderwell, in *Proven Promises*, relates the alone feelings he experienced when he underwent radiation treatments for Hodgkins Lymphoma. He says, " . . . it's a strange experience to know that everyone else will leave the room before the machine is turned on—because they know how powerful it really is. And there you are, all alone under this mega-voltage machine."[4]

What can lighten this isolation? Physical touch conveys warm feelings and affirmations of love. Holding hands while praying is helpful. It is comforting to have a friend or relative close to us as we undergo the turmoil of tests and treatments. Words can be few but just a presence there is comforting.

We also need to be able to talk to a friend, pastor, relative, or counselor about our needs. Talking may be difficult or strained at first but will become easier in time. We need you to listen. And when I dare to tell you that I'm feeling lousy, don't say, "Everything will be all right." Things won't be "all right." We have an incurable condition and we need to talk about our isolation and aloneness without you jumping in with answers to questions that cannot be answered. Don't tell us that we shouldn't feel that way and trample on our feelings.

Family members and friends are worried and concerned for us and sometimes in order not to add to their distress, we keep many of our apprehensions and thoughts to ourselves. That increases our sense of isolation.

Everyone else can run here and there, attending to their lives. But here we are at home in bed—a terrible burden to others. We don't want to take too much of their time, but we still resent them for going on with their lives. We really want to be alone much of the time, yet we want them to take care of us. We feel left out when other adults take our children shopping, to the beach, or to ballgames.

Alone

In the stillness
  of the dark night
while others sleep
I have my time alone with God.
Over the last seven years
  many people have become
  part of our lives.
  As my disease progresses
  more and more people
  fall by the wayside.
Their eyes will never
  meet mine.
I know that ultimately
  everyone
  including my family
  can leave me.
I feel alone.
I feel trapped inside a diseased body.
Yet, I know I am not lonely,
I'm just resting
  ALONE in God's hand.
—Marcia Van't Land
Summer 1987

We Feel Helpless

Journal entry of August 24, 1984: *My urine ran down and over my wheelchair again. My mom had to clean me up. I'm so filled with despair. What do I have to look forward to? More and more parts of my body giving out? More doctor and physical therapy appointments? More time spent in bed? I'm so tired, Lord. Please let me know that you care about little ol' me and my family.*

Feelings of helplessness are a big problem for us situationers. In *Still a Lot of Living: Coping with Cancer,* a woman writes, "I am deeply angry over the way patients (not only cancer patients but any patient with a life-threatening diagnosis) are automatically treated as if we were mentally incompetent. Our relatives have RIGHTS: we have none. This is by a sort of mutual consent, an unconscious conspiracy which seems to be part of our culture. Let an individual become a patient and he is treated, without any competency hearing, 'as if he had been found in a court of law to be incompetent'. Only the relatives are consulted or empowered to make decisions . . ."[5]

Although bedridden, a patient is still capable of discussing treatment options, financial arrangements, and normal day-to-day living decisions. Even if I'm in the hospital, I can still parent our children. They know they can phone me anytime, and I get calls like, "Mom, how much detergent do I put in a load of laundry?"

"Ugh." Bang, urhm, bang, bang. Those are the sounds of me opening the door at our church's educational building. The banging is my wheelchair hitting the door.

"Why don't you wait a few minutes and let me open the door for you?" asked one woman.

I replied, "But I like to do it myself."

We both laughed. I hate it when I have to ask for help.

> *People must understand that a major way to cope with fear is to remain as independent as possible.—Marcia Van't Land*

We Become Self-Centered

It is normal for a person in a chronic situation to become concerned about his aches and pains. The more uncomfortable one becomes, the more worried he is about himself. "The human mind keeps itself concerned with solving problems of living and when illness or accident comes, it poses a life problem, so that the mind turns its energies inward."[6]

Sick people often want to be alone with their pain and illness. Family members should not feel slighted when they are asked to leave the room. Sometimes sick people don't have the energy to talk or even to listen to others. That's why I prefer to be in a hospital room by myself. I have all I can manage to get myself back in shape so I can go home. I don't have the energy or time to listen to a roommate's problems. When I have a flare-up again, I'm often preoccupied so that I am hardly aware of the sights and sounds around me. I never think to have someone water my plants at home. I don't even think about what Tom and the kids are having for dinner. I have found that it is absolutely necessary to be self-centered for a time.

Sometimes our self-centeredness is actually rooted in a fear of support from others. We flee from tenderness and deprive ourselves of the warmth of life. We think that to accept love and caring is a further sign of weakness. Family members usually misunderstand someone who rejects love and goodness from them. When these types of problems occur, professional counseling is often helpful.

It's also easy to get used to pampering. It's nice to be taken care of and to shed the cloak of responsibility. This too is somewhat normal and to be expected. But we can use this as a cop-out and a means of getting our own way. I hope that if I use this means of escaping responsibility, someone will give me a friendly kick and tell me to "grow up and face reality." Please remember, though, that we do need some-one to listen to us complain now and then. We need to express our aches and pains and tell how disease is affect-ing our lives.

We Feel Hopeless

Being disabled in some way alters our ordinary sense of time. The hours and days float by as the situation in-creases and we lose hope. When we are fatigued or in pain we don't have the push or drive to do anything for our-selves. We don't have the ability to lie back and think, *This too will pass.*

Sometimes I'm just too tired and weak to hope, and then I need my friends and family to hope for me. Wounded and confused, I cower in the fear of another blow. Each time I am knocked down a piece of me dies. Why try so hard to get back up when I know I will get knocked down again? This is the time when we can discover what it truly means to be part of the spiritual body of Christ—times when others bear our burden and hope for us, have faith for us, keep going on for us. This is part of what it means to help "weaker" members of the body. "Weak" can mean spiritual deficiency, but it can mean a lot of other things, too—like just being too tired to hope anymore. The hope of others carries us while we get replenished enough to go on again.

Often my physical hope lies in having my wheelchair parked where I can see it from my bed. But I borrow heavily from God's hope. Whenever I can, I repeat the words of Romans 12:12: "Be joyful in hope, patient in affliction, faithful in prayer."

We Feel We Have Lost Our Pride

Pavel Nicholayervich Rusanov, in Solzhenitsyn's *Cancer Ward,* knows perfectly well that the ever growing lump on his neck has put him in a cancer ward. What he cannot accept is the loss of his status—he is an important official—but he quickly discovers that cancer is a great equalizer. He finds himself in a ward with eight others, all of whom he regards as social inferiors. But a new state emerges: Pavel realizes with a shock that he is not one of the milder cases.

He tries to pull rank and threatens the doctor with saying that he will inform the Ministry of Health to report the way things are conducted at the clinic. He ends up begging for treatment. Serious illness and accidents are great equalizers and can turn a man of pride into a creature of shame. No one is exempt. Nothing can buy health.

Doctors and nurses expose, examine, probe, and squeeze any part of us they choose. We feel like we are just bodies without any emotions. Robert Chernin Cantor puts it well: "Hospitalization is a single minded realm that leaves nothing for the special grace of being. Identity and uniqueness are reduced to biological anomalies, and the dramatic loss of one's identity can be extremely painful to experience."[7]

Needing help with medical expenses is another blow to our pride. People are genuinely willing to help us, but we don't want to feel indebted to anyone. Sometimes we don't have a choice as to whether we receive help; it is necessary to survival.

It bugs me when I need others to clean, cook, and do laundry. I've had to relax my housekeeping standards over the years. I keep asking myself these questions: "Is this going to matter ten years from now?" and "To whom is this activity important?" Many times I've needed help but didn't want to admit it. I appreciated people who would just back off and wait for me to decide if it would be okay to receive help. I'm learning that people don't look down on me. Allowing others to help me permits them to use the special gifts God has given them. Last Sunday at church I asked a woman to push me to the adult education program meeting. She said, "It's so nice to do something for you."

We Feel Discriminated Against

We are all familiar with the types of discrimination faced by people who have glaring disabilities—the avoidance people have for those who look different or who cannot communicate as easily as "normal" people. People in wheelchairs are still fighting for their rights and have gradually been granted such necessities as access ramps and restrooms they can enter and use.

Those of us with less obvious "hidden" disabilities face even more kinds of discrimination. "Oh, but you look so well. I can hardly believe you have a serious medical condition." Some of us are in very life-threatening situations, but we don't show it outwardly. No one knows what we've gone through in order to even be out in public. No one knows that when we get home we go to bed for the rest of the day. Often those of us with hidden conditions are accused of complaining and "putting on" when others cannot see any signs of illness or injury. Please take us seriously.

> *It takes someone mighty conscientious to tell the difference between being tired and lazy.—Unknown*

Many of us hold jobs, raise families, attend school and church, go to shopping malls, engage in sports, and do anything else we consider normal in our society.

Talk with us as you would with others about current events, sports, politics, or movies. We have likes and dislikes, hobbies and interests. We have things we can or can't do. Keep in mind that we are all hindered in some way, limited and weak before our Father.

Don't talk down to us. Most of us have learned to deal with our situations and have valuable advice to pass along. I've found that when I write a card to someone who is ill, I know what they are experiencing and am able to be very candid but encouraging.

One time three camp staff workers tried for half an hour to understand what a man with cerebral palsy was trying to say. After a while he said it wasn't important, but they persisted. "No Jim," they said, "If it's important enough for you to say, it's important enough for us to understand. Just keep trying." Finally, dozens of tries later, they got it: "The crickets sure are noisy tonight." They looked at one another and burst out laughing.

Don't be afraid to laugh at humorous situations. It won't hurt my feelings. Most people take themselves too seriously anyway. When I tell crazy wheelchair stories it makes me more of a human being. One day our children and I were out shopping. We were getting out of the elevator when the door closed on my wheelchair. I was stuck. I couldn't go forward or backward and there was no one in the elevator to push the "Door Open" button. People gawked at us, not knowing what to do. I started laughing and then they laughed rather nervously, too. I had one of the kids go over me into the elevator and push the

"Door Open" button and we went on our way, enjoying the experience.

Encourage us when we want to try something new. We may not succeed the first time—eventually we will. If we do have to ask for help, oblige us without patronizing. Doting over us robs us of our self-confidence. We need people to say that we're doing a good job at managing our condition. Tell us that we are courageous persons.

Encouragement along the Way

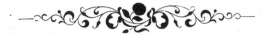

The Time Is Now

If you are ever going to love me
love me now. While I can know
the sweet and tender feelings
which from true affection flow.
Love me now
while I am living.
Do not wait until I am gone
and then have it chiseled in marble,
sweet words on ice-cold stone.
If you have tender thoughts of me,
please tell me now.
If you wait until I am sleeping,
never to awaken,
there will be death between us
and I won't hear you then.
So if you love me, even a little bit,
let me know it while I am living
so I can treasure it.
—Unknown

Part Two

Dealing with the World of Medicine

4

Doctor Who?

Cast all your anxiety on him because he cares for you.—1 Peter 5:7

Those of us involved in challenging chronic situations are dependent on the assistance of others. When we and our families are faced with declining health, intense emotions become our constant companions. Because doctors offer the hope of a cure, they take a primary role in our lives, as well as an emotionally explosive one. This chapter will focus on the doctor-patient relationship and how it can be used in a positive way.

Let's stress first of all that getting the best medical care in times of illness or accident does not mean we're denying our faith in God. God works through people skilled in the medical profession. We must pray that he will work through these skills in our particular situation, and we must view the doctor as God's instrument, rather than a "necessary evil" or some compromise of our faith.

What medicine is all about is patient care, not doctor ego.—Isadore Rosenfeld, M.D.[1]

How We See Doctors

Some people go to a doctor for help, get wheeled into a hospital, and never bother to ask questions. They just accept what the doctor says and then they die. They never try to find out about the condition themselves; they leave it all in the hands of the doctor.

One man was not told for ten years that he had multiple sclerosis. His doctor and wife kept these facts from him. I could hardly believe that story when I read it. Every patient has the right to know what is going on in his body and mind.

Who of us would give a stockbroker control of our life's savings just because he was recommended to us by a friend? Yet people entrust their bodies and lives to doctors about whom they know almost nothing. Dr. David R. Stutz says, "In no other profession that involves relationships between free adults is the authority and the decision-making power vested so heavily on one side."[2]

Do not continue to consult with a doctor whom you dislike or distrust. Over the eleven years of my illness, I've learned how to spot a good doctor, nurse, or technician when I see one. We need to remember that our doctor and health-care team members are our employees. We agree to pay for time and service. In return the medical professional agrees to give his or her best skills and knowledge. We should consider our contract with them in the same light that we would consider a contract with any other professional.

But we also want a doctor who can give us hope and confidence. He must show courtesy, respect, understanding, and avoid pretending that he knows it all. Try to find a physician who combines technical skill with a proper attitude. You have a right as a patient to make sure that your interests, concerns, and fears are an important part in deciding what treatment is best for you. Remember that it is the responsibility of the patient (or his family) to make the final decision about the use of a drug or treatment. The physician can only give you the facts and relate his experiences in cases similar to yours.

In the past, many people put their whole trust in a doctor because he generally had more training and education than most people. But with the rise of health-care awareness as well as costs, the public shares more of a responsibility and shouldn't let the medical profession call all the shots.

The chronic situationer can develop a strong feeling of faith in his or her doctor. We want to believe that the doctor's skill and power will protect and cure us. In his book *Doctors, Hospitals and Medical Care,* Richard H. Blum observes, "Having faith makes the sick more comfortable and secure in the face of the unknown."[3]

Every patient comes with his or her own "baggage"—history and orientation regarding physical and emotional problems. Many times we are in pain and confused. And we want, frankly, the impossible. We want the doctor to have no other patients before us so we don't have to wait to see him. And we want him to have no patients after us, so he'll spend time with us. We want to be able to reach him on the phone whenever we want, but we don't want him to answer other patient calls when he's with us. We want him to return our phone calls immediately.

At the other extreme is the patient who is so intimidated and awestruck by the doctor that he's afraid to ask for anything. You don't want to take much of his time because he is so busy. You don't ask all the questions you have, or ask him to repeat what you don't understand. You're reluctant to phone him even when something worries you because you don't want to disturb him. You don't dare to tell him that you want a consultation with another doctor because you might annoy or irritate him.

> *Never trust a doctor whose office plants are dead.—Erma Bombeck*

If we don't get cured, we tend to blame the doctor for the failure of our health to return. Most of the serious troubles between a doctor and a patient come about because of this disappointment. Another reason patients become discouraged with their doctors is that they come to expect too much from medicine because of the publicity in newspapers and magazines about scientific miracles and advances. Your doctor cannot use every new treatment. But if you learn of new treatments, discuss them with him or her. We want to have good health again. We want to go back to work. We want to be cured. But, for most of us situationers, the only care our physicians really can give is to treat our symptoms as they occur.

Your Medical Team

The chronic situationer needs a good ongoing relationship with a doctor that can provide easy access to office and hospital services. First of all, when we are facing a diagnosis, prognosis, or recommendation that may drastically alter the course of our lives, we need to get a second opinion. No matter how devoted we are to our doctor or how much we dislike antagonizing him we owe it to ourselves and our families to consult with another physician. Any good doctor will not take this as a personal affront.

> *The doctor's job is to educate, to advise, to counsel. The patient's job is to accept responsibility to tell the physician what works and what does not work.—Larrian Gillespie*[4]

In my case my neurologist welcomed several opinions because of the rarity of porphyria. Several times my doctor made the appointments for me to consult with other specialists.

A specialist often reads more scientific journals, is aware of newer treatments, and attends medical meetings in his specialty. This can be of much benefit and reassures us that everything available is being used for our condition. In the course of my disease I've consulted with several neurologists, interns, anesthesiologists, surgeons, gynecologists, dermatologists, rheumatologists, radiologists, family practice doctors, dentists, pharmacologists, physical therapists, a gastroenterologist, physiatrist, chiropractor, pulmonologist, and a psychiatrist. I include dentists at this point because my disease affects my gums and teeth. I can call my pharmacist anytime for information on side effects of medications I'm taking or for clarifications of prescription directions. He is an important part of my health-care team.

Even consulting with a specialist can be confusing. The medical profession does not speak with one voice on many fundamental medical questions, such as those concerning hysterectomies, cholesterol, coronary bypass, and others. Medical procedures change over the years. Some years back a person who had a heart attack was forced to retire from work and was treated with bed rest. Today coronary bypass surgery is performed and the patient is put on a vigorous physical rehabilitation program after which he returns to his job.

When consulting with a specialist, you may want to have your medical records forwarded so the specialist can read them. Other times a specialist will want to repeat all the tests in his facilities.

Consulting with a specialist for a second, third, or fourth opinion can mean consulting with another doctor in your area or some clinic or hospital in the United States or a foreign country. "The consultant should be a board-certified or board-eligible specialist who limits his practice to that specialty which concerns itself with your disease or complaint." [5] University or teaching hospitals may have top scientists who are doing research in areas that apply to your disease, but they won't, as a rule, have the time to get to know you or deal with the daily problems of your illness. But consultations with such personnel may be helpful. You may discover that your doctor was correct in his diagnosis, and that the tests and procedures in various settings have the same results.

On the other hand, the doctor in private practice may have compassion and the right bedside manner but be out of touch with the latest developments. Our choice of a primary care physician depends on our condition. If we are in remission, our medical care can be handled well by a physician in private practice. If our attacks are more frequent or a downhill slide begins, and the primary care physician has run out of ideas for treatment, then it is time to find a doctor at a university medical center.

> *You know you're involved in a chronic situation when all the names in your little black book end in M.D.—Marcia Van't Land*

Coordinating all the medical data from various specialists is important but difficult to do. It's very important that you have a primary care physician who can oversee your medical care. He will be the one you see most often and who monitors your medication and general health problems. However, a specialist can also serve as the primary care physician. For a five-year period my neurologist served as my primary care physician. I now have an internist serving in that capacity. In most HMO's the patient is required to consult with a primary care doctor first. He must give authorization before additional services can be rendered or an appointment made with a specialist or a therapist.

Practices vary in terms of what particular services you can expect from your primary care physician, depending on his expertise. Another aspect to consider is whether your doctor has hospital affiliations and what and where they are.

> *Most doctors recommend the procedures that are most likely to result in the longest survival, without as much consideration for what they see to be more tangential issues: possible pain or discomfort, disfigurement, loss of function or independence. Many physicians are far more comfortable talking about survival or life extension—issues that are relatively quantifiable—than about such subjective issues as "quality of life."—David R. Stutz* [6]

When my diagnosis was conclusive and I didn't want more diagnostic tests and procedures, I concentrated on finding a doctor who wouldn't feel threatened by my knowledge of my disease. I needed a physician who would be part of my health-care team and feel comfortable with the fact that I would never regain my health. Yet I wanted a physician who would help me live in the most productive way possible. For example, he recommended that I have a hysterectomy in the hope that we could stabilize my hormones. When my badly diseased bladder would no longer function, he recommended that I have it removed. Both of these procedures helped stabilize my porphyria.

How Physicians Feel

Doctors hate disease and accidents as much as we do. They feel powerless because they know that no treatment is going to stop the progression of the condition. We underestimate how much our doctors care about us and how often they discuss their cases with their colleagues. It's like getting a free consultation and it greatly benefits us.

Dr. Jane Patterson, in her book *Woman Doctor,* relates how terrible she felt when a deformed, dead baby was born. On the outside she remained as unemotional and professional as possible. She says, "when death wins, the doctor has lost, and doctors, perhaps more than most people, don't like to lose; death is a personal affront."[7]

Physicians also fear death in the same fundamental way we all do. "I didn't know what to do or say or how to behave with a dying person. That wasn't included in medical school curriculum in my day. . . . These women were dying and I was terrified of their deaths. . . . My terror of these deaths was all entwined with my terror of my own death. I kept my distance."[8]

In *Head First,* Norman Cousins talks openly about the heavy weight of responsibility that doctors carry with chronic and terminal patients. He functioned as a counselor and doctors would refer their patients to him so he could "give them courage and hope, to bolster their will to live and to try to lessen the depression that so often accompanies a serious diagnosis." He goes on to say, "But the steady progression of patients in the terminal stages of illness cuts deeply into my consciousness. . . . If it were not for the occasional case that comes through despite overwhelming odds, I doubt that it would be possible to move on to the next patient."[9]

The doctor may have a hectic schedule and he didn't get enough sleep the night before. He may be concerned about personal problems. "He needs to feel helpful and of value to you. If your condition gets worse, in spite of everything he does, he feels frustrated, helpless and inadequate. He wants to be liked, respected and appreciated by you, just as you want to be thought well of and cared for by him." [10]

Bedside and Other Manners

We do need to realize that many doctors are overworked. Doctors also have to prepare themselves to do all sorts of things over and above the call of duty. Sometimes they must mediate a disagreement between patient and family members. They can get involved and end up being a marriage counselor. Medical schools and young physicians try to stay clear of these functions, but older doctors know that the "extra" comes with the profession. Even so, the one complaint mentioned often by patients is the lack of compassion from the medical profession.

Many medical schools are revising curriculum to have their doctors develop more awareness and compassion for patients. At Harvard University Medical School, the curriculum was rewritten four years ago to include communication skills as well as scientific knowledge. The students must meet regularly with patients during the first week of classes—not, as in years past, in their third year of medical school. The students regularly meet with chronically ill persons. One of the benefits of particular meetings was to note that often in the cases of chronic situations, the supporting spouse and family need encouragement and care also. Other medical schools require that doctors work at a homeless shelter and become acquainted with an elderly patient.

In a Los Angeles Times article entitled, "Learning Bedside Manners," the point was made that "medical groups and educators are paying more attention to how doctors communicate with their patients. Some physicians are finding out what it's like to be hospitalized. Wearing backless gowns and hooked to I-V's, they learn firsthand the sense of helplessness endured by patients."[11]

Howard Markel, M.D. wrote an article entitled, "Remembering Debby," where he related how his young wife died from liver cancer in spite of the new procedures. He says, "Once I could only understand my patients' reactions to grave diagnosis. Now I know how they feel." He goes on, "Anxious to save the world, I found going to work each morning was exhilarating. But I quickly noted the stress associated with telling patients their diagnosis." He notes how his relationship with a patient changed after announcing bad news. He felt horrible for all of them and for having to be the one to tell them they had a deadly disease.

Now that his wife, Debby, had incurable cancer, he was on the receiving end and looked at the doctor with feelings of hurt, disbelief, and even anger. He concludes the article by saying, "And now, when forced to present bad news to patients, I find it useful to remind myself how it felt to receive it."[12]

Hollywood has even picked up on the bedside manner issue in the movie *The Doctor*. A hotshot surgeon is a great surgeon but an arrogant snob. When he develops throat cancer himself, he learns that there is more to being a surgeon than cutting.

Doctors also admit that there are patients who have survived serious illness not because of medical treatment but because of a powerful will to live. Most doctors have seen medical miracles that can't be explained. God can still perform miracles when he chooses.

Being a Good Patient

The chronic situationer sees his or her doctor frequently, so the relationship tends to be more personal. "In addition, well-informed patients who are managing chronic disorders, such as diabetes, Parkinson's disease, cancer or AIDS are more likely to keep abreast of the latest research about their problems or may belong to peer support groups in which current information is exchanged." [13]

It is easier to come to grips with a chronic situation if we replace our ignorance with information. We humans have an amazing capacity to deal with situations if we know what we're dealing with. We become fearful of the unknown but medical knowledge helps us take better care of ourselves.

Many times we can get medical information from pamphlets the doctor has given us, but if we want more information, a trip to the library is the best road to take. Many library reference departments have access to medical literature via computer, and most librarians are happy to help you. I have found that purchasing my own *Prescription Drug Encyclopedia* and a *Medical Encyclopedia* to be very helpful. It was three years before I connected with the National Organization for Rare Disorders, Inc. (NORD). Their literature has been great and I list their address in the hope that more chronically ill persons will be helped: NORD, New Fairfield, CT 06812. NORD has information on over five thousand rare diseases and a referral to appropriate sources of assistance.

Somehow, the doctor and the patient must communicate and make decisions about the patient's health care. They must move from their own perspectives enough to meet on common ground and understand the real enemy, which is the disease itself. Here are some suggestions for the person who wants to be a "good" patient.

Have an agenda—a specific purpose—for each office visit. You need a general plan for the things you want to tell the doctor and the questions you want to ask the doctor. Are you concerned about some side effects from a medicine you've been taking? Are the side effects worth the positive aspects of a drug? Are there developments in the way you feel or are reacting to present treatment that you need to bring to the doctor's attention? A doctor learns from the way you present your concerns. Studies have shown that when patients ask forthright questions, they receive better medical care. By now my doctor knows me well enough that he'll ask if we've covered everything on my list.

Insist that your questions receive answers. Vicki Goldish, executive director of the Wellness Community, a cancer support group, doesn't waste words. When she developed cancer five years ago, her surgeon informed her that she had cancer and abruptly left the room. She called him back, looked him in the eye, and demanded a full explanation.

We have the right as patients to ask questions and expect answers. Don't be afraid to ask the doctor to write down specifics when he is giving you instructions for change in diet or medication.

Be honest about your symptoms. Present the facts. Don't be "strong" and say you are doing fine when in actuality the pain and the weakness are worse. A doctor cannot help a patient who doesn't give complete information.

Have a friend or relative with you during doctor visits. Particularly if you are not feeling well, another person can help you sift through what happened during the appointment and keep your information straight.

Be sensitive to technical medical terminology. There have been times when my doctor used language I didn't understand. I immediately asked him to clarify the information he had just given me before we went on to other matters.

Some of us in chronic situations and especially those of us who have rare or orphan diseases may know more about our disease than the doctor does. This can be a touchy subject and I try not to come on strong with technical medical terms. I try to remember that the purpose of this office visit is not to prove who knows the most about my disease. I need my doctor to guide my path and help me maintain my condition as well as we can for as long as we can. It is a partnership.

Establish a good working relationship with the doctor's office staff. The receptionist and nurse screen the phone calls before you can get through to the doctor. If your doctor says you can call him anytime, don't abuse that privilege. Don't make every symptom an emergency. Give a new symptom (unless acutely painful) two or three days before calling. Most of the time, it can at least wait until office hours.

Be prepared when you call the physician's office. How you present the facts on the phone to the nurse usually makes a difference in whether you'll get through to the doctor.

Be aware that you may have to wait a week or more to get an appointment. If you are an established patient you can usually get in more quickly.

Try to be a patient patient. Waiting in a reception room or in the examining room can be frustrating. Much of that frustration could be prevented by better planning. If you know you have a doctor appointment for 11 A.M., don't make plans to meet a friend for lunch at 12:00. Emergencies come up regularly for a doctor. I was impatient during the earlier years of my disease. Then I had two times in which I was the emergency and kept other patients waiting because I needed immediate attention. I try to keep things in perspective.

I've also found it helpful to take my own writing, reading, or craft materials along. Then I don't feel that my time has been wasted. Friends or relatives usually bring me to a doctor appointment and we use the waiting time to talk and update each other.

The waiting room can become a window to life's problems. I see the various forms and colors of those who are ill or injured. An Alzheimer's patient—sixty years old—walks all over the couches and pillows in the waiting room, as his wife frantically tries to control her husband's behavior. A ten-year-old girl sits in her wheelchair with her limbs contorted from cerebral palsy. Seeing others' pain helps me keep my own in perspective.

Illness and accidents may rain down on the just and the unjust alike, but good patienthood can be learned and is a must for situationers. A positive relationship with our medical support team is necessary. Each time we need medical attention, there are many witnessing opportunities. Sermons are preached without saying a word. We must make certain that we are giving God's message to others—through our patience, our kindness, our willingness to keep trying, to have faith. We can, with God's help, turn a lousy situation into a positive one.

Encouragement along the Way

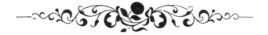

*T*he best recourse for you is to try to keep abreast of those advances in medicine of particular relevance to you—not in the posture of challenge, criticism or suspicion, but with the spirit of partnership, which is what a good patient-doctor relationship is all about.
—Isadore Rosenfeld, M.D.[14]

5

You and Your Hospital

He who dwells in the shelter of the Most High will rest in the shadow of the Almighty. I will say of the LORD, "He is my refuge and my fortress, my God, in whom I trust."—Psalm 91

For many chronic situationers, hospitalizations become a substantial part of medical care. Many of us have spent long, lonely, and painful nights in unfamiliar and often frightening hospital environments. At the same time, hospitalization can provide a warm and caring place in which we can find healing and relief from pain.

We have reason to be proud of medical resources in the United States; we have impressive research capacities, cutting-edge technology, and a good system of medical education. Unfortunately, that does not mean that each person will get the best care from a doctor or hospital. Only when we take responsibility for our own care and insist on high-quality care from medical professionals can we expect the best results.

It is important that you exercise some control over your health destiny. Getting the most out of medical care does not come naturally. It must be learned.

Choosing a Hospital

All hospitals are not equal. Some are better equipped to treat your particular condition than are others. Unfortunately, important information is not always obvious, and an ill person seldom has the time or energy to comparison shop. There are some factors to consider when it is time to choose a hospital.

Size and location. There may be two or three hospitals in the immediate area, and you should know what type of care each of them offer. There are two kinds of hospitals: the university or teaching hospital/medical center, and the community hospital, which is usually a smaller facility. Community hospitals vary widely in the care units they provide. The university or teaching hospitals generally are affiliated with a medical school program and often can provide highly specialized care.

It is helpful to talk to friends or relatives who may offer valuable advice based on their personal experiences with local hospitals. Your doctor or the local nursing association is another source for information.

The nature of your medical problem. Someone who has had a heart attack needs immediate medical attention and will not have time to go to a distant hospital. If your condition or illness involves extremely specialized care, you may be willing to travel to a hospital equipped for your needs.

Your physician's hospital affiliation. Is your doctor on staff at the hospital of your choice? You may have to switch doctors in order to receive the best overall medical care.

Health insurance limitations. Will your health insurance cover hospitalization in the hospital you choose? Some health plans are only in force in certain cooperating hospitals and clinics. In the past, some health insurance policies refused to pay for certain diagnostic tests unless the patient was in a hospital. Now insurance companies insist on day-in-day-out procedures, saving them money.

The tendency among doctors to hospitalize a patient only when necessary has become quite common. Many insurance companies call the attending doctor each day a patient is hospitalized. The doctor must justify that the patient needs to be in a hospital. And insurance companies want details, not generalizations.

Health-care Systems

When asked, "What is the state of health of our nation's health-care system and can we cure it?" the former Surgeon General of the United States, Everett Koop, said, "Our health-care system is in crisis, bordering on chaos . . . changes that are needed are so complex that it will take us a decade to get from here to there."[1]

People fear what a serious illness or accident would do to their pocketbook if they needed a serious hospitalization or outpatient treatments. They worry that if they require medical care they will lose their insurance coverage. Chronic situationers are often stuck in dead-end jobs because they may lose their health insurance when they switch employment. Some insurance plans will not cover a pre-existing condition or will raise the premiums so high that no one can afford them.

It is estimated that thirty-seven million Americans have no health insurance at all. Some are eligible for assistance from the state or federal government, but it is difficult to find a doctor or a hospital that will treat them for the limited fees Medicaid will pay.

Many people do not know what health insurance coverage they have until it is too late. Insurance plans are dull reading, but it is important to understand your coverage. Nearly everyone experiences the expense of illness or accident in some form or another. And the older we become, the more health care we will need.

Health plans available

Service plans are run by two nonprofit organizations, Blue Cross and Blue Shield. They pay hospital and outpatient charges. There is usually a deductible required.

Commercial plans pay a fixed sum for medical services. The insured person is responsible for all charges in excess of these indemnity amounts.

Health maintenance organizations (HMO) are called "prepaid" plans. There are no "deductibles" and no "maximums" but the insured can only use member doctors and hospitals. The organization receives a fixed amount for services. They have various rules and coverages and need to be investigated thoroughly.

Medicare provides insurance for a physician's services and hospitalization for citizens who have reached sixty-five years of age. Many people eligible for Medicare need to buy additional private health insurance because Medicare only pays about half the expenses.

Medicaid is a combined federal- and state-administered program that pays for medical care for welfare recipients such as the disabled, the blind, and families with low income and dependent children. Each state has its own program.

Social Security disability should be investigated to learn whether you're eligible or not. Call your nearest Social Security office to obtain the forms you need to complete.

While investigating an insurance plan, it is important to determine your deductible, the cost sharing plan, and the exclusion plan. Voluntary services, such as cosmetic surgery, may be excluded. Other policies do not cover specific diseases, conditions such as organ transplants, or mental illness. Also be aware of the "caps" on your coverage. A "cap" is the highest amount the insurance company will pay on a certain condition.

In dealing with medical insurance companies, it is important to keep copies of the bills and claims, as well as an accurate record of all your transactions and payments. Since many insurance companies are large corporations, and you may go through several persons and offices in one conversation to get information, it's a good idea to keep track of names of persons as well as the titles for their departments.

Although insurance companies were originally intended to provide financial security for people during times of illness and injury, some of them have become quite shrewd in their methods to avoid paying out large sums of money. They rewrite plans and change benefits offered without informing policy holders of the changes. Or some have been known to drop policy holders who became big financial risks.

The health insurance industry is bound to go through change, since many Americans—as well as their representatives in Congress—have declared that the high costs and endless bureaucracy have become unreasonable. While health-care bills are thrown around at all levels of government, chronic situationers and their families need to make sense out of the policies they presently have. Stay in close contact with your private insurer. The Social Security office can also provide some information. Don't keep concerns to yourself; during these times of possible change more people than ever are needed at the local, state, and national levels to make known the needs and views of people in chronic situations.

Life in the Hospital

People go to the hospital because they believe they will have a better chance to survive, since doctors have access to modern technology and expert nursing care. But hospitals are not familiar environments; they can be quite intimidating.

Be an informed patient. You may not be able to change basic routines, but at least you can understand why these routines are necessary. You should know whom to call when a conflict arises and how to effectively lodge a complaint.

In a sense, patients own the hospitals. You pay for them through your medical fees, your insurance, your taxes, your church, and your community efforts. The hospital is your territory, so it only follows that you should know it fairly well.

Admissions

Admissions to a hospital can be done by pre-admission or on an emergency basis. Obviously if it is an emergency, much of the admission procedure changes and accelerates. But you must have the following information with you: Social Security card, insurance cards, Medicare and/or Medicaid cards, information on your employer or your spouse's employer, name/address/phone numbers of person to notify in case of emergency. This is also a good time to give the nurse a card listing your current medications and dosages; this will save you having to answer even more questions.

A new law requires every hospitalized person to sign an advance directive or living will—we'll talk about these documents in chapter 12.

Daily routines

The daily routine in any modern hospital can involve a great deal of pain. Every day, and sometimes more often, lab technicians come into your room uninvited to draw blood. Many diagnostic tests and treatments are uncomfortable, if not painful, and on top of that, they can feel quite degrading. How is a person to survive all this?

You must remember that your first priority is to get well enough to be able to go home. Sometimes it helps to focus on an upcoming event and remind yourself of the purpose of your life. A loved one or a nurse holding your hand can get you through the pain of a spinal tap, bone marrow test, or mylogram.

Know the details of your hospital agenda and what is planned for you on a day-to-day basis. Then you'll be in a better position to avoid the mistakes that can happen. For instance, many tests and procedures are performed early in the morning before the doctor arrives, so it is a good idea to ask the nurses about the purpose of the test, when it will occur, and what the conditions are. Often a patient is scheduled for a test that requires no food or drink after midnight. The breakfast tray may be delivered anyway. If you eat or drink, the test must be postponed another day.

Always read the Informed Consent form before signing it. It is your insurance company or you who will be paying the bill, and the decision to complete the test or not is yours.

Know your medication schedule and check the dosages before taking any medication. It has happened to me several times that a nurse brought in the wrong medications. *You have the legal and ethical right to refuse medications.* The nurse writes, "Patient Refused" on the chart and later you can discuss this issue with your doctor.

If you have an ostomy, prosthesis, or any other medical condition that is not related to your current hospitalization, make sure the nursing staff knows how to care for it. I have a urostomy and take all my own supplies with me to the hospital. When it needs to be changed, I talk a nurse through this procedure. Do not assume that all hospital personnel are knowledgeable about all procedures.

The role of nurses

Your best assurance for a tolerable hospital stay is to develop a good relationship with your nurses. If you treat them with respect and courtesy, you are likely to get courtesy and respect in return.

The care of hospitalized patients is a constant, twenty-four-hour-a-day process, and most of the responsibility for that process rests squarely on the shoulders of the professional nurse. She is there when a patient's heart stops beating in the middle of the night. The nurse informs the patient of what to expect in certain tests and procedures. The nurse monitors the basic needs of the patient and communicates with doctors and the family. She becomes the confidante of seriously ill or injured patients. Dying patients need to express their intimate emotions, and often it is the nurse who shares these moments.

> *NURSES: Credible Professionals Doing an Incredible Job—bumper sticker*

"Each year during the month of May, a week is set aside as *National Nurses Week.* All across the country hospitals, nursing homes, visiting nurses associations, doctor's offices, rehabilitation facilities etc. take this prescribed week to recognize the indispensable role the professional nurse fulfills in insuring all citizens, no matter their health related problems, obtain qualitative health care services."[2] Nurses deserve recognition.

The nursing staff can help the patient by offering guidance, advice, and the encouragement to keep going and progressing. They can quietly allow the patient to assume more responsibility in his own care. They can stimulate the patient to renew his interest in the world, make plans for the future, and convey hope. Staff members may talk with the patient and suggest he become part of a support group to learn from others in similar situations.[3]

Know your rights

As a patient, you have the right to:

- Request to read your hospital charts. Your chart is a complete record of communication between members of the hospital staff, and it documents all of their contacts. Many physicians and hospital staff feel that a patient should not read his chart. They maintain that information on the chart may upset some patients. You also can misinterpret information found in your chart. On the other hand, patients who reviewed their charts on a daily basis said that it helped them understand the nature of their progress.

- Give informed consent prior to the start of any procedures and/or treatment.
- Refuse treatment.
- Insist that all communications and records pertaining to your care should be treated as confidential.
- Refuse to participate in research projects.
- Examine and receive an explanation of your hospital bill regardless of source of payment.
- Leave the hospital at any time—even before the course of treatment is finished. (The only exception is patients who are committed to a hospital psychiatric unit on an involuntary basis.) If you decide to discharge yourself against your doctor's advice, inquire if your insurance would cover for services rendered. Some insurance companies refuse to assume financial responsibility for a patient who signs himself out.

Maintaining your equilibrium

You can survive the hospital stay, even though much of it may be unpleasant. Draw upon your own spiritual resources, first of all. When in pain and facing difficult decisions, repeating God's promises over and over will help you feel a closeness to him. During a difficult time I would repeat, "I can do everything through him who gives me strength" (Philippians 4:13).

Talking to a chaplain, other hospital personnel, friend or relative may be helpful. Perhaps your relative may say that he really misses you at home and is looking forward to your homecoming. That in itself can rejuvenate your purpose for the day: to do what needs to be done here (in the hospital) so that you can return home.

This may seem to go without saying, but don't worry about your hospital appearance. You feel terrible and look that part, dressed in a drab hospital gown, your hair stringy. This isn't a beauty contest, and visitors don't expect you to look wonderful.

> *Most people do a lot of looking up when they are lying down.—Granger Westberg*

Be aware that your health problem needs to be dealt with immediately, but also remember that your family still needs your love and concern. You haven't stopped being a spouse, a parent, a child—a family member—because you are hospitalized. Your family is having a tough time, too. They need any emotional support you can give them.

Feelings of isolation and frustration can really pile up during a stay at the hospital. Having large amounts of unstructured time can cause a lot of stress. You have so many emotions inside and you can't go golfing to get away from it. Your medical condition is constantly there and time passes slowly. You wonder how things are going at work and at home.

Try to maintain a link with life *outside* the hospital. Have your family bring reminders from home. Ask questions about the weather, current events, and family life. If it's possible, have your children visit often so you can keep up with their lives. It is important for children to see their loved one in the hospital. Not only does it lessen their unnecessary fears about what you are going through, but it helps them see for themselves why you are not home with them—that you really are ill and have not deserted them.

Many hospitals allow a family member to stay with you. They provide cots or fold-out chairs for no extra charge. Having a family member spend the night can alleviate much of the fear and apprehension that come with hospitalization.

Cultivate a sense of humor. In chapter 7, we'll talk more about the benefits of humor. I have found that when hospitalized, anything on the lighter side is welcome.

Finally, in the excitement of returning home, it's easy to forget certain instructions and prescriptions. Keep a list of your questions so that when your doctor signs you out, he can answer them. Have the doctor write out any diets, prescriptions, or treatments. Instructions can quickly become jumbled otherwise ("Was it two of these pills with every meal, or am I supposed to take two a day, but make sure I eat before doing so?") If the patient is faced with an altered lifestyle and role, the social service department of the hospital should be informed. They should schedule a family conference in which the needs of the patient and family are discussed.

Medic Alert

Most of us don't have hospital personnel around us all the time who understand our condition. Sometimes our health crises occur away from home and far from the doctors and nurses with whom we have become so familiar. We must be careful to fill in the gap of information in the event that we require unexpected treatment.

Tragic, even fatal, mistakes can be made during emergency medical treatment if hidden conditions are not recognized. For this reason millions of people wear the Medic Alert emblem as a bracelet or a necklace. On the back of the emblem is engraved the patient's medical condition, such as diabetes, asthma, or allergies to drugs such as penicillin. This small metal disc will speak for you if you can't. Emergency and health-care personnel are trained to look for it.

Also engraved on the emblem is a special "call collect" number that provides instant access to your emergency medical records and the names of physicians or relatives to be contacted. This twenty-four-hour emergency answering service is on call every day of the year.

Medic Alert members also carry a wallet identification card that contains additional personal and medical information.

For more information, write:

Medic Alert Foundation International
P.O. Box 381008
Turlock, CA 95381-9008

A Question of Treatments

Most chronic situationers have tried various treatments and procedures with success in some and failure in others. Well-meaning friends and relatives will offer information and suggestions. Sometimes that turns out to be a real help; other times you have reached yet another dead end.

There are four basic categories of healing: natural healing—the body heals itself, arguably the most frequent kind of healing; medical healing—the physician assists the body with various medical treatments; "quack" healing—the unproven claim to heal the body on the basis of false or questionable methods; and divine or spiritual healing—God heals the body. Many medical doctors attest to cases in which the cure was unexplainable in purely medical/scientific terms.

Chronic situationers can be very susceptible to anything that will improve their physical health. They desperately want to feel better and their emotions and feelings often override their intelligence.—Unknown

The kind of medical establishment that we are accustomed to in the United States evolved during the middle of the nineteenth century and is considered both "traditional" and orthodox medicine today. The prevailing opinion of this establishment is that the most practical ways of combating disease rely on drugs and surgery.

Homeopathic practitioners and natureopathy methods are still very much alive in the Unites States. *Homeopathy* uses minute doses of substances that produce the same symptoms as does the disorder. This form of treatment is known to have no real effect in the treatment of disorders. *Natureopathy* is a therapeutic system in which natural agents such as fresh air, exercise, and massage are preferred to drugs or surgery. Conventional drugs are not used. The medical establishment considers these methods unproven and unorthodox.

Much has been written in the last few years about the New Age Health Movement. New Age medicine can be described "as the modern practice of diagnosis and treatment by a medically unqualified and often psychically oriented practitioner using methods for which effectiveness has never been established or has been scientifically discredited. Even when a practitioner is medically qualified, this does not validate a new age treatment. . . . those who practice new age medicine do not usually have the medical skill of a regularly trained physician."[4]

Especially at a time when health-care costs are unmanageable and the public is losing its trust in the medical community's desire to heal over the ambition for monetary gain, it is very tempting to turn to "new" kinds of treatment. In the case of New Age practitioners, "new" is often a revival of very old methods, methods that the medical establishment either knows little about or has explored enough to deem ineffective or unreliable.

So what is legitimate practice and what isn't? To help us determine this Dr. David Sneed and Dr. Sharon Sneed have written *The Hidden Agenda*. Drawing from years of investigation and documented case studies, the authors write about more than 25 alternative medicine treatment methods. This book is available in Christian bookstores.

Medical Miracles and Research

Any of these headlines sound familiar? "Virus Raises Hope for MS Vaccine; One Last Chance—Ovarian Cancer is Killing Young Women; Conventional Treatments Have Failed—Their Life Depends on an Experimental Therapy That Would Block the Action of a Deadly Gene; Looking for Small Miracles to Extend Life Even One Month; Blood Breakthrough Could Aid Immune Systems; Medical Research Saved My Life—Coulbourne's Tumor Disappeared After a New Drug Regimen; New Laser Technology Cleared a Woman's Blocked Coronary Arteries; A Research Drug Helped a Woman's Severe Rheumatoid Arthritis; Vaccines Against Colon and Kidney Cancer and Melanoma Are Being Widely Tested; Miracle Medicines Coming Our Way."

While some such announcements may be fluffed up for publicity, they attest to the extensive work being done to find breakthroughs that could prolong or save lives and conquer disease. Any chronic situationer should stay abreast of current research in the area of his or her condition. You don't want to miss out on anything that could help you. And there is usually too much new data being generated for your doctor to know everything about your disease.

Before any drug, vaccine, or medical device is approved by the Food and Drug Administration, it must go through a process of extensive testing. In the first stages, studies are restricted to animals. Then if the experimental therapy is safe and shows promise against a certain disorder, human trials progress.

There are pros and cons for being involved in a new therapy. Researchers are testing the new treatment for any advantages it may have over existing approved therapies. If the treatment appears to involve great risks, it is stopped. On the other hand, if a treatment is proving valuable, others involved in the program will receive that new treatment.

It's possible that you will be approached at some point about participating in medical research. Be aware of the aspects that need to be explored.

Before volunteering for research, ask—

1. Who is sponsoring the research? Trials could be sponsored by a major health organization, drug company, the federal government, or a university.
2. Will there be pain or discomfort? What kinds of tests will be involved? Find out the answers before you sign a consent form.

---

3. Who monitors the trial? Who makes sure that this trial is legal?
4. How often will you need to be examined? What if you live far from the research center?
5. Will your doctor get a record of the results? The attending doctor should be kept up-to-date throughout the trial.
6. For what other condition can this research be helpful? What has been the record of safety?
7. How much will it cost for you to test this drug? Will you continue to receive the drug if it is approved? Most companies will offer the test drug to participants for free.

Orphan Drugs

Orphan drugs are the large number of effective, safe medications that have been rigorously tested and licensed in other countries outside the United States. Sometimes approval in the United States can take up to nine years.

In 1983 the Orphan Drug Act was passed, making federal financial assistance available to "pharmaceutical companies, individual researchers, nonprofit organizations for the development and marketing of some drugs previously unavailable in the U.S. One aspect of this law is to accept drug studies from other countries so studies do not need to be repeated in the U.S. Also an individual American citizen can bring a reasonable quantity of an orphan drug from another country for personal use."[5]

Don't hesitate to inquire about orphan drugs. The world of medical science is quite miraculous, and it is peopled by doctors, nurses, technicians, and researchers who care very much for those who are ill. Sometimes they must distance themselves from patients because they face so many hurting patients in a day's time; they have a need to protect themselves emotionally. But, overall, hospitals and the people who staff them are aiming to help you get well. They are looking for answers, too. To them it's a huge battlefield, and they want to win against disease.

When you turn to doctors, nurses, and hospitals, you entrust your health to others. Keep in mind the bigger picture of living as well as you can, looking at your whole life, and cooperating with those who would participate in your healing.

> *Jesus Christ checked into this big hospital. He became a patient just like the rest of us. He suffered more than we do. The more we learn about his suffering, the more help we get when our faith is tested by hospitalization.—Marcia Van't Land*

Encouragment along the Way

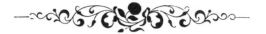

*T*o Hospital Personnel
Here are some *bravos* for you, from hospital patients:

- "The nursing staff showed a lot of concern for me."
- "I really appreciated the care of the nursing staff when I was in a great deal of pain. The nurses listened and did not make me feel guilty when I complained."
- "The people in physical therapy were fantastic. The aides who transported me there were very uplifting. It really helped my morale."
- "I appreciated it when my nurse would check on me periodically even when I didn't call her."
- "The nurses stayed in touch with my doctor and informed him when my condition changed."

But here are some words worth remembering:

- "The staff didn't seem concerned enough about my discomfort, and often I had to wait an unreasonable amount of time for pain medication. Nurses tried to tell me that I wasn't in as much pain as I said."
- "Doctors and nurses don't give satisfactory answers to patients' questions. They're always in a hurry."
- "Doctors should ask patients, 'How are they treating you? Is the staff courteous? Anything you need?' "

- "Lack of privacy and noise pollution really got to me. My sleep was interrupted. The canned music nearly drove me bananas. The hospital has no right to impose their noise on patients."
- "I think the patient should be told exactly what medications they are being given and why."

6

Chronic Pain

*If I rise on the wings of the dawn, if I settle on
the far side of the sea, even there your hand
will guide me, your right hand will hold me
fast.—Psalm 139:9-10*

Pain is the primary reason for most doctor visits, and the treatment of it costs our economy close to $90 billion annually in medical expenses and lost productivity.

Pain is an important defense mechanism. Pain can tell you if you are overusing an injured joint or are interfering with the natural healing of a sprained ligament. People with Hansen's disease (leprosy) have damaged nerve cells, and when they touch something hot or sharp they feel nothing. God created us with pain receptors for good reasons, but when we experience pain we often need help in dealing with it.

Pain is many things to many people. It is no respecter of persons. One of the most frustrating aspects of pain is that it cannot be measured, pictured, or truly understood by anyone except the person experiencing it.

> Patient: "Doc, it hurts when I do this."
> Doctor: "Then don't do that."—*A classic vaudeville joke*

Acute Pain

Ordinary or acute pain "yields to medical treatment or to the body's own superlative healing apparatus within six months."[1] Acute pain serves a purpose. It is a warning signal that something has gone wrong with your body. It is a message from your mind to take action to remove yourself from danger.

All pain can be excruciating, but with acute pain, each day the pain becomes less. Even when the pain is intense you know you are on the mend.

Chronic Pain

Chronic pain exists over time. Any pain that stays longer than six months is termed chronic.

Chronic pain is *not* part of the healing process. In fact just the opposite is true. With arthritis the pain is a sign of active disease or of its crippling consequences. Chronic pain often seems to have no meaning; it is unpredictable and intermittent. It can be sharp or dull, stabbing or boring, crampy or steady. It can stay in one location or move. Those in chronic pain can rarely predict when the pain will let up or recur.

"The National Institute of Health estimates that chronic pain afflicts at least 90 million Americans and counts among its victims those who suffer migraine headaches, back pain, arthritis, trauma, and catastrophic illness."[2]

For some people, pain is a way of life. If you're a victim of chronic pain you know that no one else can comprehend your discomfort and frustration. Pain is experienced alone; it cuts you off from others and can make your body feel like a prison.

There is a "fellowship of those who bear the mark of pain." Those without pain—outside the fellowship—have great difficulty in comprehending what lies behind the pain.—Albert Schweitzer

If you let chronic pain consume your life, it will. "For too many pain sufferers, the list of things that it hurts to do expands daily until it includes most of the activities in their lives. Brick by brick, the prison walls rise."[3]

The mechanism of pain is subject to great misconceptions by patients and physicians alike. In his book *Toward the Conquest of Cancer*, Dr. Edward J. Beattie, Jr. states that "pain is controlled poorly by many physicians in the United States and thousands of patients suffer needless pain, which is a medical disgrace."[4] Chronic pain sufferers and the medical profession need to work together on this important issue.

Questions to Consider when Consulting a Physician about Chronic Pain

1. Where exactly is the pain located? Is the pain worse when moving or unchanged with positions?
2. What does the pain feel like? Sharp, dull, steady, stabbing, burning?
3. On a scale of 0 (no pain at all) and 10 (the worst pain imaginable) tell the doctor the score for this pain.

---

4. Does anything you do make it better or worse?
5. What other symptoms are you experiencing?
6. Have you experienced this pain before?
7. Have you taken any pain medications and did they take the pain away?

The best way to treat pain is to treat the illness. Unfortunately, there are some chronic conditions where the pain never seems to ease up, but a bit of compassion and concern on the part of a caring doctor can sometimes make those pains a bit easier to bear. Physicians are not always able to fix underlying problems.

Pain is mediated by sensory nerves that pass through the spinal cord on the way to the brain. "Most pain originates because of irritation or pressure on the tiny nerve fibers that end in the skin or underlying tissue. It can, however arise from pressure or inflammation of the nerves itself, even at the spinal cord."[5]

Only certain tissues of the body are capable of "feeling" pain. For example, people with lumbar disc problems can tell about referred pain—their back condition causes serious pains down into the leg. The brain itself does not "feel" pain but the structures that cover it do.

Some people are more sensitive to pain than others. A difference in nervous system functions and of the presence of endorphins in the brain can cause wide disparity in pain tolerance.

Pain Treatment Centers

In the last fifteen years a new medical specialty has been developing. Pain centers—both inpatient and outpatient— are springing up throughout the country, as chronic pain specialists attack the problem from many angles.

Therapy may include biofeedback, acupuncture, nerve blocks, hypnosis, autogenic training, group therapy, medication, physical therapy, nutritional counseling, and many others. Not all centers offer the same approaches to pain relief. What these centers do is try to conquer unnecessary, intense pain and help the patient establish coping mechanisms. There are more than thirty conditions that can cause chronic pain. It is not just a medical problem, but an interrelated emotional, social, and familial problem.

Most medical centers and hospitals offer pain management techniques. These programs are expensive but many insurance companies cover the costs.

In the early 1980s I spent three weeks as an inpatient at the Portland Pain Center. Their manual listed four highly specialized skills that would be taught there: 1) to learn pain control and coping skills; 2) to eliminate use of narcotic analgesics; 3) to improve physical and emotional functioning; 4) to increase self-reliance in pain-related health care.

"By the time a person has lived with pain for months and even years, a number of negative effects are likely to have appeared. Not only does the person suffer the immediate effects of the pain itself, he or she also has begun to feel the impact of painful disability upon emotional functioning, family life, vocational capabilities and recreational interests. These tend to accumulate, from reduced physical capacities, long-term use of powerful analgesic medications and a general loss of positive activities in daily living. The suffering person and his/her family are often overwhelmed as more burdens are added."[6]

Learning chronic pain behavior at the PPC was a multidisciplinary approach. Available to the patients were physicians, psychologists, registered nurses, physical therapists, occupational therapists, a social worker, and a biofeedback specialist—all experienced in treating pain problems.

There were also lectures on the physiology of pain, time management, interpersonal relationships, job and stress management, disability issues, assertiveness training, and diet.

Family members were strongly urged to participate in learning what would be helpful in maintaining the gains from the program.

Methods for Coping with Pain

Here are some brief descriptions of techniques currently in use for dealing with pain. Each person finds the technique(s) that works best for him or her. Often a combination of techniques is most effective.

Relaxation

Head-to-toe relaxation exercises can be learned and are very helpful to relieve accumulated stress and tension in your body.

Deep breathing is the simplest and perhaps oldest of the total relaxation techniques. Close your eyes. Make yourself comfortable. Breathe in—deeply . . . from your diaphragm. Then breathe out . . . slow and easy. When you are relaxed, your heart rate and blood pressure drop. Blood flows to the brain and the skin rather than to the muscles. Your rate of breathing and your consumption of oxygen decline and your brain waves shift to a relaxed rhythm. The result is that you feel warm, rested, and mentally alert.

In a Relaxation Session we would lie on mats and, using pillows, try to make ourselves comfortable. The whole purpose of these sessions was to relax enough that we wouldn't feel the pain.

We had a retired physician in our group, and one day halfway into our session, he fell asleep and started snoring. We tried to continue, but soon I could hear snickers coming from all over the room. That ended *that* session!

Biofeedback

In biofeedback, you are hooked up to a monitoring device that gives evidence of how chronic pain is affecting you. It also shows the control you can have over pain.

The goal of biofeedback training is to teach you to reduce tension and therefore pain by giving you information about the internal working of your body (e.g., muscle activity, skin temperature, and perspiration).

Guided imagery

At the center of our being is the "eye" of the soul, a vibrant, vivid, incredulously powerful mechanism called imagery.—Richard M. Linchitz[7]

"The western world's health care establishment has only recently acknowledged imagery as a valid and valuable technique for the management of chronic pain, even though imagery has been in use for centuries as a primary element in the disciplines of yoga, meditation, hypnosis, and psychotherapy."[8]

More specifically, guided imagery can be created and directed for the therapeutic purpose of relieving chronic pain. In guided imagery it is helpful to associate your pain with subjective imagery. For example, I imagined the pain in my abdominal, lumbar, and hip areas as cement. Then I imagined Ms. Pacman eating up that cement, keeping time with the beat of my TENS unit (Transcutaneous Electric Nerve Stimulation).

TENS

Transcutaneous Electric Nerve Stimulation is the passage of small electrical currents through the skin for the purpose of controlling pain. Electrodes are placed over the site of pain or along the nerves innervating the area. The patient operates the control, making the shock sensation strong but not uncomfortable. The major problems of the TENS are irritation or soreness of the skin under the electrode, and the inability of some patients to learn to use the device. Then there's the problem I had. While wearing a TENS unit, one pad fell into the toilet, and I received a good shock.

> *When I turned sixteen I had to learn to live with chronic pain and to understand that it will always be there. I have tried to live my life free of pain, but this illness has me fighting the toughest battle of my life.*—Ruth Pecor[9]

Physical therapy

The purpose of physical therapy is to teach you how to improve body alignment, increase mobility, strength and endurance, and to improve your understanding and use of body mechanics. Usually there is an evaluation time to distinguish what your specific physical problems are and to set realistic goals.

Physical therapy often includes a scheduled pool therapy in which the patient participates in a series of general flexibility exercises designed to improve the range of motion, endurance, posture, and body mechanics.

Posture and body mechanics classes also teach how your anatomy and posture can affect different parts of your body. These can be applied to your lifestyle.

Occupational therapy

The role of occupational therapy centers around the disruption in a person's ability to live a meaningful life due to chronic pain. Occupation means being occupied in meaningful day-to-day activities including work, play, and leisure. Usually occupational therapy is primarily concerned with the effect that pain can have on your lifestyle and activity, what activities you choose to be involved with, and how you use your body in these activities as a means of pain control.

Occupational therapy teaches how to use your body in non-stressful ways, working smarter, not harder, pacing yourself, and applying good body mechanics. It often includes vocational counseling and/or rehabilitation.

Distraction

By using diversion, a person's attention can be focused away from pain. This method can take various routes. Some people can distract themselves from pain by imagining themselves in a fantasy situation far removed from where they actually are. One woman spends hours in extended daydreams based on novels she likes to read.

A person can get outside himself by watching TV, listening to music, talking with others and learning more about their lives, or getting busy with an enjoyable activity. Caring and thinking about others takes your mind off yourself and your pain.

> *Most important, you need to change your viewpoint . . . to an abiding focus on other persons or on constructive activities. You must get that black spotlight off yourself.*—Dr. James Kenny

I have found that focusing on a beautiful poster of a field of tulips can divert my attention away from my pain. I picture myself bending down to smell the tulips and walking through narrow aisles separating each variety. I concentrate on the color and style of each section and think of how much work it must have been to plant so many.

Setting short-range goals for each day can motivate you to put your pain farther back in your mind. Feeling needed by others also helps you to concentrate on something besides your own struggles.

Aim for being as independent as possible. This will improve your self-image, thus enabling you to focus on what you can do rather than on what you can't do.

Pharmacology

To take or not to take—that is the big question. Drugs can be an extraordinary help in coping with pain, but they need to be seen in the broadest context. Drugs are only one tool among many in the realm of pain control. Many over-the-counter drugs can be effective in relieving mild or moderate pain but are not effective for every person with chronic pain.

The pain was just terrible, so terrible that you are not yourself anymore—you are pain—everything in the world is pain. Sometimes more particular than that: you are impaled by it, unable to escape. Racing with pain, trying to escape into the gas while the tongues of pain lick at your heels, like the tide overtaking you.—Anne Morrow Lindbergh[10]

The issue of narcotic drugs for chronic pain remains an emotional one, and people are quick to take sides or jump to extreme positions. Many doctors say, "Painkillers for chronic pain—absolutely not. If aspirin doesn't do it, try gritting your teeth."

The drug companies say, "You have pain? Relieve it by all means."

Some of the non-narcotic drugs like anti-inflammatory agents are helpful. Those with chronic pain often become depressed, and there are many drugs that can ease depression.

"In our drug-conscious society . . . with the social abuse of drugs and the stigma of drug addiction, there is an understandable but unfortunate apprehension among both patients and physicians regarding the legitimate use of narcotics to relieve pain."[11]

A September 22, 1991 issue of *The Los Angeles Times* states that "Nancy Reagan's 'Just Say No' anti-drug campaign and the Bush Administration's 'get tough' attitude on the illicit drug trade may or may not have had an effect on the use of street drugs. But it has undoubtedly affected medical care in hospitals, for it has made doctors even more fearful than they already were of addicting their patients." [12]

The latest, more scientific studies show that opiates are not addictive when given for real pain. "The most widely cited of the recent studies in 1980, found that only four of

11,882 hospital patients who had no history of addiction became hooked on narcotics during treatment."[13]

Dr. Jamie Von Roenn of Northwestern Memorial Hospital in Chicago recently found that 85 percent of cancer specialists surveyed acknowledged undermedicating their patients. The vast majority rarely even asked patients about pain.

A sixty-year-old man with bowel cancer spread throughout his body had so much pain he couldn't eat, walk, or even sit without suffering acute discomfort. At night he would awaken every two hours, screaming in agony. He was pleading for his life to end until he visited a new oncologist. This doctor was appalled to learn how little pain-relief medication the man was receiving and prescribed morphine.

The next morning this man's wife found him preparing breakfast, and for the first time in months he had slept through the night. The medication couldn't save his life, but it certainly improved the quality of the life he had left.

Addiction has become such a highly charged issue that pain specialists are using the terms *drug dependence and tolerance* instead.

"It is essential that patient and physician understand that tolerance and physical dependence do not imply drug abuse . . . the person receiving a drug for relief of pain is quite different from the person we know as a drug addict who is both psychologically as well as physically dependent on the drug."[14]

The questions remain: "What is quality of life? When does 'better living through chemistry' begin and end? What is the alternative to using pain control drugs—suffering?"

New developments in pain control

The last few years have seen some exciting pharmaceutical developments. These more powerful drugs have fewer side effects and also a new technology for delivering those drugs into the body at lower dosages. For example, "Epidural catheters can be inserted near the spinal cord to deliver morphine or other medications that block pain from reaching the brain. There are also new bandage-like patches to deliver painkillers through the skin, and long-acting narcotics that need only to be taken once a day for continuous pain relief." [15]

For the pain after surgery the computerized Patient Controlled Analgesic pump, in which the patient pushes a button to medicate himself from his hospital bed, uses less medication and results in shorter hospital stays.

In 1986 a group of health professionals in Wisconsin initiated a program to transform cancer-pain attitudes and care in their state. The initiative included:

1. "Advocate the teaching of cancer-pain relief in medical and nursing schools.
2. Inform patients and their families that pain can be managed.
3. Examine drug laws to find out if there are legal barriers to proper cancer-pain management.
4. Make clear that fears of addiction are overemphasized." [16]

Now more than seven states are considering similar programs such as the Wisconsin program.

Coping with Continuous Pain

Many readers of *Accent on Living* responded to their poll question: How do you handle chronic pain?

One person has been living with pain for forty years. She says, "Over the years I have tried many things. Really the best thing is having a good doctor who understands and believes you when you say you can't handle it anymore and gives you pain shots. I do my best to forget about the pain by distraction."[17] She uses medication until she brings the pain under control enough to use distraction methods.

> *Nothing slows a clock like pain: Nothing speeds it up like keeping busy.—Sefra Kobrin Pitzele*

Some people in the poll said they just live with the pain. Others use exercise, rest, meditation, water therapy, or hot showers, acupuncture, TENS units, ultrasound, surgery, self-hypnosis, medications, massage, and relaxation. Still others use trigger point blocks, cortisone injections, yoga, visualization, imagery, and chiropractors.

> *Someone would say, "My, you look well today. I'm glad you're feeling O.K." I would think, If only you knew. No one understood enough to share my burden. What a lonely thing pain is—a very personal thing that others cannot understand unless they've been there too. Instead of understanding I often received rejection.—Dorothy Snell*[18]

Only 30 percent of the *Accent* respondents had tried a pain clinic. Some found it helpful but one person in particular had a very negative experience.

The results of the poll show that people are dealing with pain the best way they can. Pain management is not magic and it takes hard work and discipline. You may never be pain-free, but the pain can be eased and take its place in the back of your mind.

Learning about our pain and how it affects us makes it less scary. So learn all the methods of pain control mentioned in this chapter and give them a try more than once. Some only work if you keep trying.

JoAnn Kelley Smith says in her book, *Free Fall,* that "one's personal relationship with God and the reality of Christ's presence do not eliminate all physical pain. We still must handle the anger and depression that chronic pain brings into our lives." [19]

Tim Hansel talks of his eventual surrender of daily physical pain after years of praying for healing. He says, "I finally came to the realization that if the Lord could use this body better the way it is, then that's the way it should be." [20]

We situationers need to come to the point where we can accept our chronic pain as part of our lives and go on from there. Again Tim Hansel says, "I have prayed hundreds, if not thousands of times for the Lord to heal me—and he finally healed me of the need to be healed. I had discovered a peace inside my pain." [21]

Remaining embedded in our own little world of pain gets us nowhere and drives people away. We have no choice. We can do nothing but endure.

> *If I say, "When I am strong, then I'll be joyful," "When the pain eases, then I'll be joyful" . . . if I'm going to wait until I feel like it, I'll never do anything.—Marcia Van't Land*

Even while we are in the midst of pain we need to learn to be content in our circumstances. Often when I'm in intense pain, I am unable to pray. That's where my family and friends come in. They pray me through another difficult episode and I can feel Christ's presence within me. In that sense I have accepted my pain and can say, " I have learned to be content whatever the circumstances" (Philippians 4:11).

Learning how to handle chronic pain may be the toughest challenge you face in this life. By gaining some control over it, you will feel more in charge of your life and more positive about living with your illness.

Encouragement along the Way

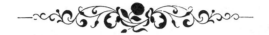

Guests

Pain knocked upon my door and said
That she had come to stay;
And though I would not welcome her
But bade her go away.

She entered in, like my own shade
She followed after me,
And from her stabbing, stinging sword
No moment was I free.

And then one day another knocked
Most gently at my door.
I cried, "No, Pain is living here,
There is not room for more."

And then I heard His tender voice,
"'tis I, be not afraid."
And from the day He entered in—
The difference it made!

For though He did not bid her leave
(My strange, unwelcome guest,)
He taught me how to live with her.
Ah, I had never guessed.

That we could dwell so sweetly here,
My Lord and Pain and I,
Within this fragile house of clay
While years slip slowly by!
—Unknown

7

Emotional Health

*Be strong and take heart, all you who hope in
the* LORD.*—Psalm 31:24*

A common response to the news of a serious diagnosis is
sadness or depression. The chronic situationer cannot help
it, but his condition leaves him hopeless and despairing of
ever returning to health. He loses confidence in himself and
in the future. When people face a loss or a challenging
situation, they say, "Well, at least I have my health." Now
we can't say that.

Those of us who have chronic situations in our lives are
at a higher risk for depression and stress-related illnesses.
The normal pressures of life are compounded by dealing
daily with a situation that will never go away.

When I began having serious health problems I was
scared. Nothing was the way it should be. What will happen to me? How long will I live? Will it be painful? What
can be done medically? Will our insurance pay the medical
bills? Will people stop loving me and abandon me? What's
going to happen to our children? What if I can't take care
of myself?

I frantically tried to hold onto the fact that I could still
walk with a cane. Every time I was hospitalized I came
home so weak that I needed a wheelchair to get around the
house. After a few days I would relegate the wheelchair to
the garage, vowing never to use it again. Gradually I

needed the wheelchair more, and without us realizing it, the wheelchair was becoming part of our family. This in itself was depressing.

Sadness and depression have a number of causes. Chronic illness and accidents are the only ones we will deal with in this chapter. It is also important to distinguish between a full-blown clinical depression and the state of being in a "down" mood. Lucille Kulper, in her article, "Journey from Desolation," makes this observation: "To compare 'feeling down' to the illness of depression is like comparing a small paper cut to major surgery."[1]

A grim diagnosis is quite enough to erase a smile and plunge one into despair. Depression often occurs when sickness and death are both seen in a patient's mind. When my friend, Cathy, received the diagnosis of inoperable liver cancer, she felt as if the whole world had crashed and was covered with a black cloud. The sun didn't shine. The flowers and people were distorted and she had no idea of how to cope with life and the situations it might bring. She would wake up at night and be terrified. She would repeat the words of Psalm 91:4-5: "He will cover you with his feathers, and under his wings you will find refuge . . . You will not fear the terror of night." Often in depression the patient has changes in sleeping or eating habits. He experiences irritability, anxiety, and fear. Changes in his body as a result of medication or treatment can make him self-conscious. God may seem far away and silent. Some medical conditions can stimulate depression: "hypothyroidism or adrenal and pituitary abnormalities, multiple sclerosis, brain tumors, lupus erythematoses, some vitamin deficiencies and infections such as hepatitis, flu, and mononucleosis."[2]

An August, 1991 associated press article in the *Inland Valley Daily Bulletin* stated that clinical depression affects nearly ten million Americans and is often more disabling than arthritis, ulcers, diabetes, or high blood pressure. Depression can limit people not just in emotional ways but also physical ones. It can cause problems with walking, dressing, bathing, climbing stairs, or participating in sports. Coronary artery disease and heart pain are the only chronic conditions that are more disabling than depression.

> *Being happy is just about the hardest of all activities.—Nathaniel Branden*

Treatment of depression is a major challenge. Approximately 20 percent of those who are depressed actually get treatment; the majority suffer in silence or are misdiagnosed. Often depressed people will be told that their problems are too much tension or anxiety, a personality disorder, or weak character. Whenever people are involved in a chronic situation, they are very susceptible to depression. They may have feelings of hopelessness they are unable to shake. *Why go on and try so hard when I know this disease is going to kill me anyway?* That type of thinking is normal— but should only be temporary.

Be familiar with the warning signs of depression:

- Change in appetite or sleeping patterns
- Low energy level
- Sad and hopeless feelings
- Inability to concentrate
- Agitation or irritability
- Withdrawal from others
- Sexual problems
- Thoughts of death or suicide

Steps to Take When Depression Strikes

At the onset of depression you can do the following:

1. Recognize your need for help. Talk to a valued friend or relative about your depression. He or she can give support, listen, and suggest possible solutions. If what you come up with doesn't help and the depression doesn't lift, don't hesitate to seek out the expertise of a trained counselor or therapist.

2. Talk to God if you can. Take all your burdens to him. That doesn't mean just shooting "arrow" prayers like "please help me to have a bowel movement—today if possible." It means taking all our fears and insecurities, all our doubts and habits, all our individual and family situations to the Lord. If it helps, talk out loud to God. Some people find it easier to write down their thoughts and feelings. Sitting at the computer and typing a prayer to God works, too. The method isn't important as long as you know that God does listen and answer.

In Psalm 38:21-22, David cries: "O LORD, do not forsake me; be not far from me, O my God. Come quickly to help me, O Lord my Savior." God will enfold you with his loving arms and give you rest. There may be times during which you can't pray. This is normal and God understands. It is a good idea to have a trusted relative or friend pray for you and with you.

3. Evaluate your physical condition. Is there any physiological reason for your depression? Make a doctor appointment if necessary.

Check any medications you are taking. Tranquilizers, sleeping medications, antihistamines, or painkillers may be affecting you emotionally. Several times while I was hospitalized we stopped all my regular medications, and depression followed. One of the reasons this happened was a drop in my level of female hormones. After a few days of resuming these hormones, my depression lifted. If you suspect that any medications are causing your depression, give your doctor or pharmacist a call and get information.

4. Try a change of scenery. Be as active as possible and include new activities or hobbies to give you a positive boost. The chronic situationer must realize that his or her condition contributes significant stress to the situation. At other times it can help a depression if you eliminate activities that cause you anxiety. Saying "no" is not easy but is sometimes necessary to your health.

5. Get as much physical exercise as possible. I taught physical education from kindergarten through high school for a number of years and I know the benefits that exercise can bring to body and mind. In the early stages of my disease, I tried various workout programs. The first time I went to a water exercise class, I tried to keep up with the class. The next day I could hardly move. I discovered that three repetitions for each exercise was all I could handle. No matter what restrictions you have you can usually carry on *some* level of activity.

6. Make decisions and don't look back. Indecision can frustrate. Be content with the fact that you are doing the best you can with what you have. Often chronic situationers must make decisions regarding their course of treatment. Once these decisions are made don't say, "Well, maybe we should have done it this way instead." Hindsight is always 20-20 vision. I have found it helpful to write down all the options that are available. Seeing those options in black and white make decisions easier.

7. Take charge of your future. Chronic situationers may feel that life is beyond their control. Set short- and long-range goals. Work toward reaching these goals. An example of a short-range goal: "If I can only get three loads of laundry finished, the day will not have been a waste."

A man was told by his doctor that he had thirty days to live. He said, "If I only have that much time to live, I'm going to enjoy it." Earlier, before this news, he had drawn blueprints of the addition he wanted to put on his house. So he ordered the necessary materials and went to work. Twenty years later he is still alive. I don't know how large his house is by this time, but the point is made: If chronic situationers have long-range goals, they live longer and are happier.

8. Reach out to others. Doing this will put you one step beyond your own needs. Isolation can drive you deeper into depression. Studies have shown that getting "outside" yourself stimulates the immune system. Even a phone call or writing a note to someone who is ill can be a positive thing to do. Don't just lie in bed or sit in front of the TV. Force yourself to walk around the block or call a friend.

9. Let yourself cry. Tears can physically and emotionally wash away our fears. When I feel sad about my disease and the losses it brings, I go into our bedroom, shut the door, and cry until there are no more tears. My eyes get red and puffy. My nose clogs and my voice becomes hoarse. Then I try to sleep and put everything out of my mind. When I emerge from the bedroom, my family is very kind and loving to me. They know that I have again worked through all the trauma that comes from being in a chronic situation.

10. Increase your laughter. Joke about the mundane things in life. Try not to take yourself too seriously. Concentrate on enjoying your family and friends. Studies have shown that smiling at least once an hour can be beneficial to your mental health. One woman asked her husband, "Why are you smiling at me?" He replied, "It's my hourly smile."

> *We must be joyous over the things that can be and not despair about the things that can't be.—Marcia Van't Land*

11. Seek out a support group that pertains to your situation. This group can be formal or informal. Much can be learned from outside speakers. The very act of putting yourself in touch with others who are also chronic situationers can help you work through problems. More on support groups comes later in this chapter.

12. Seek outside and professional help if the depression continues for more than a few weeks. Your doctor or pastor can usually recommend a counselor. Many Christians prefer that their counselor also be a Christian. Sometimes medications will be prescribed to help deal with the depression. This treatment should involve biological, psychological, and spiritual elements.

After coming through a deep depression, Lucille Kulper wrote, "I was struck with the thought that coming out of a depression is like putting on the glasses of the soul. What was hazy becomes clear, what was distant becomes close. I felt alive with sudden delight, surprised by the joy of my rebirth from the emotional death of depression."[3]

Depression is serious—it is costly both professionally and personally—but in most situations it can be treated successfully. With the help of friends and family a miracle will happen if we "hang in there." The world will once again be beautiful. The sun *will* shine again.

More about Humor

One of the steps that chronic situationers and their families and friends should evaluate is what place humor has in their lives. Being able to laugh at yourself and your weaknesses is a must. A sense of humor does not mean that a person is always laughing and smiling and making jokes. "Humor is first and foremost an attitude—almost an attitude toward life, a willingness to accept life and to accept ourselves 'with a shrug and a smile' with certain lightheartedness."[4]

> *No living creature can laugh except man. Trees may bleed when they are wounded, and beasts in the field will cry in pain or hunger, yet only I have the gift of laughter and it is mine to use whenever I choose. Henceforth, I will cultivate the habit of laughter.—Og Mandino*

Humor has a way of breaking life up into small pieces so you can deal with it. To lighten up is good advice for all of us; feelings can have a powerful impact on our health. Emotions can tear people apart or they can heal relationships.

Humor is an individual matter—what is funny to one person may not be funny at all to someone else. But humor is definitely contagious. One funny comment leads to another, and before you know it everyone close by is laughing—and some don't even know what they're laughing at!

> ## *Ha! Ha! Ha!*
>
> Receptionist in a urology clinic answers the phone, saying, "Urology—can you hold?"
>
> Patient with an arrow sticking out of his rear end: "Don't take it out yet—the insurance company says I have to get three estimates."
>
> Five men are crammed into one hospital bed. One guy says, "Next time I take out a group policy I'm checking the fine print."

In the study of humor—called humorology—researchers have found that when a person laughs, he or she enhances respiration and helps to oxidate the bloodstream, washing out irritating carbon dioxide. Laughter also increases relaxation for up to forty-five minutes. The harder you laugh, the more tension you release—and the longer the effect lasts. After you've finished laughing, your pulse rate drops below normal and your muscles become deeply relaxed.

Laughter is a form of internal jogging; it exercises the lungs, stimulates the circulatory system, and increases oxygen in the blood. Your chest, stomach, and face get a vigorous workout. When you really laugh hard, even your leg and arm muscles work.

> *Trouble knocked at the door, but hearing a laugh within hurried away.—Poor Richard Jr.*

In his book, *Anatomy of an Illness,* Norman Cousins tells how ten minutes of hearty laughter gave him two hours of pain-free sleep. Against all odds he made a complete recovery from a crippling disease. The former magazine editor is now a professor at the University of California, Los Angeles, School of Medicine. Humor has become so respectable that soon laugh therapy will be standard practice in health care, higher education, and even the corporate board room. Laughter is natural, free, and there's no chance of an overdose!

> *An optimist is a person who laughs to forget; a pessimist is a person who forgets to laugh.*
> *—Anonymous*

Tips for building your sense of humor

- Build a comedy collection. Jot down jokes, poems, riddles, stories, puns, etc. that look on the lighter side of life.
- Write your own "funnies"—keeping track of the humorous happenings in your and your family's life.
- Surround yourself with people who help you laugh and who find humor in the

most unusual experiences. Your family must develop their sense of humor, too. Because of complications in my bowels, I need to use a powerful laxative. The kids always tease me about my "dynamite pills" working.

- Practice your sense of humor even when you don't feel like it. Successful humor comes with doing. Find ways to laugh. Relate some embarrassing incident in your life. See if you can make someone laugh out loud.
- Develop your own personal "theme." I collect frogs and always say, "Eat a live frog in the morning and nothing worse can happen to you all day." When I'm in the hospital, our kids always bring me Kermit the Frog to hang on my bedframe He has gone with me on every hospital stay. People see Kermit hanging there and know I'm visiting again.

Support Groups

According to the National Institute of Mental Health, half a million mutual-help groups in the United States deal with almost every human problem.

Most mutual-help groups have the same purpose: to provide emotional support and practical help in dealing with a problem common to all members. There is a special bond among people who share some of the same experiences. When someone says, "I know just how you feel," it brings a sense of relief. Then your pain can be shared with the group without explaining all the minute details. Each mutual-help group should provide an atmosphere of acceptance. This will encourage its members to share their frustrations and fears and help them find effective coping mechanisms.

Any meeting of two or more people with a common interest in their situation can be called a "support group." Here are some guidelines for making your group more than a forum for small talk.

1. Establish some ground rules. Many groups agree among themselves that what is shared with the group is never repeated outside the group. Confidentiality is important. Some groups decide that certain areas are off-limits for their discussions.

2. Appoint a leader. One person may lead all sessions, or the leader may change from session to session. But unless someone takes responsibility for the direction of the discussion, it can go off in every direction or become a gripe session.

3. Determine your goals. Why are you meeting? If your goal is to discuss the weather and current events, that can be done elsewhere. Learning from your chronic situation and being willing to help others through difficult times should be the goals of each meeting.

4. The group need not be formal. Some groups meet weekly in restaurants or homes; others meet once a month. Larger groups often have officers, rules of order, by-laws, and newsletters. Join the type of group you feel most comfortable with.

5. Make speaking optional. Many people are afraid to express their feelings in a group. The larger the group the more difficult this becomes for some. In our group of seven, we take turns updating each other on the happenings since we've met. While each person speaks we all listen and then can interject comments and suggestions.

6. Some groups encourage spouses, friends, caregivers, or anyone closely affected by your condition to attend meetings. Other times caregivers need a break from their chronic situation and don't want to attend. Be flexible.

7. Be on the lookout for new therapies or treatments that may help you or someone in your group. If your group is large enough, invite outside speakers. Specialists can offer a variety of useful approaches and are willing to share their knowledge. Members of the group may be willing to read useful books and give reviews of them.

8. Make meetings special in little ways. Meet over lunch or dinner. Take some time to pray together or have a minute of closed-eye silence. This helps focus the group.

9. Some groups socialize with one another at picnics or at other gatherings. Not all people have the time, energy, or commitment for this.

10. Make sure you are "ready" to meet face to face with others in your situation. Disease and injuries are variable. Those with the same diagnosis can be affected differently. What you see or hear at support groups is not necessarily the way your situation is going or will develop in the future. You will have your own version of your situation, not someone else's.

> *God gives us the ingredients for our daily bread ...*
> *but he expects us to bake it.—Unknown*

Tears in Bottles

Psalm 56:8 (RSV) says: "Thou hast kept count of my tossings; put thou my tears in thy bottle! Are they not in thy book?" In some ancient cultures they used tear bottles when visiting a suffering friend. In this little bottle you could tenderly catch your tears as a symbol of your loving willingness to share their suffering. Often these tear bottles were kept as a memorial to having shared another's suffering in love. God does that, too. He's not offended or embarrassed by our tears. Quite the opposite. He is moved to compassion by them.

> *Another's tears are salve on our wounds.*
> *—Nicholas Wolterstorff*

Don't be afraid of tears. They are not a sign of weakness. They are a sign of strength. Your tears tell others that you are facing the realities in your life.

Likewise, those who would support you should not be afraid of tears—yours or theirs. Their tears demonstrate their care for you, that they hurt when you hurt.

Tears also act as a natural cleanser to the body and soul. Crying can remove chemicals that build up during emotional stress. Tears can make you feel better both physically and emotionally. Tears have a way of putting life in perspective. They help put your loss in a special place so that you are free to go on with your life.

Remember too that each person grieves in different ways and times. Be patient with yourself and others and learn to listen to one another.

When we are hit with depression, anxiety, or general sadness, it becomes a bit difficult to pick ourselves up "by the bootstraps," and I would never minimize the effects of emotional pain and how hard it is to get beyond it. But our overall outlook on life can still be our choice, and a healthy attitude better prepares us for tough emotional times. Make a list of behaviors in your life. Then evaluate which ones are the most important and give up the ones that drag you down. Get rid of old worries and fill yourself with new plans for a happy future.

Take part in sports, entertainment, games, hobbies, and wholesome fun. Give up any "old baggage" and concentrate on a new outlook. It's never too late to change our attitude toward life.

Encouragement along the Way

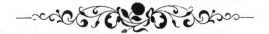

*T*hen There Will Be No More Me

My three hydrangea bushes that I ordered last summer,
   came in the mail during my last hospitalization.
Oh, I had big plans when I ordered those plants!
I could imagine how I would use their large multicolored
   flowers in floral arrangements for church and at home.
I was counting my blooms before they blossomed.
God had other plans for me and my hydrangeas.
Each time I lost one more thing, it felt as if a part of me
   was being ripped out.
The part of me that wanted so badly to live and associate
   with the living—like my hydrangea bushes—was
   being slowly taken away.
Then there will be no more me!

For a few days the open wound of the giving up of my
   hydrangeas was bitterly sore.
The wound was aggravated when our Bible study group
   went Christmas caroling in a convalescent home.
I strummed my guitar as a friend pushed me in my
   wheelchair.
Some of the residents sang and walked with us.
Others were in wheelchairs like me and were alert and
   knew the carols.
Still others sat strapped in their chairs,
   unaware of the Christmas singing.

One of the "more alert" residents shook my hand and
mistook me to be a resident there.
Then there will be no more me!

How long before the horrible consequences of this
disease will reduce my body and my mind to a blob
strapped in a chair unaware of Christmas singing?
"No Lord! Not that, please! Take me home to be with you
before that happens!"
The Lord answered, "Were you not blessed and touched
by the response of the rest home residents?
Didn't you feel that the staff at that home were loving
and kind to both residents and visitors?
Weren't you amazed that one old woman thought it so
precious just to kiss you?
Weren't you blessed by the eighty-five-year-old woman
who was blind, had a broken hip, but yet praised
the Lord?"
Then there will be no more me!

"My will and desires will become yours, O Lord.
Who am I to question how I will live and affect others?
Will you come to sing for me, hold my hand, and talk
to me?
Will you show you care by listening to my prayers?"
Yes, then there will be no more me!
—Marcia Van't Land
December 1983

Part Three

A Lifestyle of Coping

8

Becoming Overcomers

"For I know the plans I have for you," declares the LORD, "plans to give you hope and a future."—Jeremiah 29:11

The key to coming out on top of a chronic condition is simply "hanging on" and working through the acceptance phase of grief. Eventually we will arrive at the place where we can say, "I will accept my chronic situation; now I'm going to see where I can go from here without letting it run my life."

Keep in mind that acceptance will come and go. Even when we think we have accepted our situation, we will experience anger and depression from time to time. These feelings are normal.

> I jokingly say, "I have a Ph.D. in life and survival. Ph.D means 'patient hasn't died.'"
> —Marcia Van't Land

The loss of our health involves intricate changes in our lifestyle. We must deal with the discomfort and symptoms of our illness or injury and manage the stress of our chronic pain, treatment procedures, and hospitalizations. We need to get along with the medical profession so we can get the best treatment available. We have to maintain our family and friend relationships despite the possible role changes.

We may have to give up the control of our bodies. Medications or treatments may change our body image and affect our self-esteem. We constantly live with an uncertain future in which further loss, death, or recovery are all possibilities.

Humans are the only living beings that can exercise choice. No matter how disabled we are, we do have options. We are not specks of dirt being blown in the wind. We are more like snowflakes, created by God. Each of us was born for a specific reason and purpose. When God's plan for our life is completed, we will die. It is up to us to try to make a positive contribution and do what needs to be accomplished.

In the course of a chronic situation we can rant and rave to God about the unfairness we've experienced. We can try to put our heads in the sand and temporarily forget it. We can drown ourselves in self-pity or anger until it is too late. We can demand attention and become invalids long before it is necessary. We can make life miserable for our loved ones. Or, we can get the best help available to us. We can have the courage to function in whatever way we are capable and touch many lives by our valiant struggle.

A chronic situation slows us down and plunges us into the process of reevaluating our lives. We may ask ourselves, "What have I done with my life so far, and what am I going to do with the time I have left?" This decision is ours and we are wise to pray each day, "Dear God, let me not downplay the value of what I have to give. Someone else may be watching—and you are, too."

> *Health is not a stable condition of soundness throughout, like a steel building on a concrete foundation. Health is a state of balance maintained by perpetual adjustments to forces within and without.—Arnold Hilt*

Educate Yourself

If we know what to expect from our illness or accident, we can deal with it better. We can spend time in a library or get information from our doctor. Humans can deal with almost anything as long as we know what it is. When we understand our situation, we can stop blaming ourselves or others.

Keeping a journal can be extremely helpful in recovery work. We journal perhaps to record our personal history, memories, and feelings. During times of reading we might jot down flashes of insight. Beginning each journal entry with the date helps us focus and record our current inner journeys. We need not worry about our grammar and sentence structure. It is important to get every thought recorded. Rereading my journals at a later time impressed upon me how God had gotten us through some tough times and that he would certainly get us through this present crisis. We journal not so others can read it but because it helps us work through our feelings.

Sometimes it also helps to read inspirational books about how other people have dealt with and adjusted to their chronic conditions.

Recognize the Role of Stress

"Stress is a normal response to the demands of everyday life. It's a form of energy in itself and is neither good nor bad."[1] Stress can also include "frustrating circumstances, time pressures, family and other relational problems, financial difficulties, disappointments, heartbreaking circumstances, physical problems, and other situations that result in strain, pressure, or tension."[2]

Each person has his or her own response to stress. Each of us chooses whether or not we will dwell on the negative or the positive; sometimes it's necessary to think about the negative in order to work through real fears and problems—times when being "positive" is something like whistling in the dark. There is such a thing as "good" stress. Good stress keeps us motivated to live each day in a positive way. The stress of going to work and of caring for our families are examples of good stress.

Unfortunately, people who live with a chronic situation year after year acquire much negative stress. We often experience the pressure to try hard in order to show people how well we are coping—when on the inside we aren't coping at all. Stress and anger, particularly when they are repressed, can cause depression, insomnia, ulcers, headaches, and many other ailments. Add those symptoms to the major illness or accident that has occurred and we have acquired quite an overload of negative stress.

> *The real voyage of discovery consists not in seeking new lands, but in seeing with new eyes.*
> —*Marcel Proust*

Often we cannot control circumstances in our lives, but we do control how we react. *Our coping responses will either increase or decrease our stress.* We may need to change the habits we've acquired over the years. Certainly we must learn new and improved ways of coping.

There are numerous tools for dealing with stress—everything from simple deep breathing exercises to psychotherapy. Sometimes medication is required; many people hit crisis times when their bodies need an extra something to help them reclaim equilibrium. It's important to remember that being put on medication (such as an antidepressant) does not mean you will be taking it forever. It does not mean you are losing your mind. Any good physician is not interested in glossing over real problems by keeping the patient sedated. It's most important that you are aware of what stress is doing to you so that you can deal with it in the manner most appropriate to your situation.

One Day at a Time

Injury or illness comprise just one common category in the causes of stress. When a separation or divorce, death in the family, job loss, or any other life changes occur, we need to sit back and evaluate how we're going to handle them.

One of the biggest mistakes we can make is to try to do everything all the time. We'll burn out quickly with that approach. Make a simple plan for each day. Focusing and narrowing our alternatives to one day or one hour at a time can go a long way in reducing stress. Life becomes manageable when it's broken into do-able segments and tasks.

Because I realize how close to death I was several times, I am thankful for each day and usually greet it joyously. What I do with my time and energy is important. I'm learning to sort out what is really valuable and I say no to some commitments without feeling guilty about it. I'm constantly asking myself, "Will this matter ten years from now?"

For instance, I know that attending our kids' sporting events and programs is very important. I can hear them saying, "Remember how Mom would sit under a blanket with just her nose and eyes visible, so she could see our soccer games?"

> *No matter what our diagnosis, we need to enjoy*
> *common moments as well as memorable occa-*
> *sions.—Marcia Van't Land*

Orville Kelly founded "Make Today Count" after he received a grave cancer diagnosis. At first he had spent a lot of time in bed—even though he was able to walk and drive. But he worked through his feelings of possible death, fear, and isolation and discovered that he "wasn't dead yet."

Sometimes the future is so uncertain and scary we can easily spend all our time and energy worrying. When a condition is progressive we often worry about the day when we can no longer take care of ourselves. We live under the shadow of a recurrence or a flare-up. We must learn to live each hour of each day and not let the uncertain future bother us. We must try not to get all bent out of shape over minor matters. Thomas Merton reminds us that "God does not ask us to feel anxious, but to trust him no matter how we feel."

Basics of Physical Care

It should go without saying that it's important to get enough rest, eat well, and exercise regularly. Many people are lazy in matters of basic health; until they become ill they can get away with it. A chronic situation makes necessary physical care even more urgent a matter. When we are under the stress that comes with illness or disability, our bodies have special needs. We require more calories. In many cases we need more sleep and nourishment so that our healthy cells can overcome the diseased ones.

If we don't get enough sleep or are not eating correctly, we will have less ability to deal with our situation. We may have to swallow our pride and ask our doctor for help in these important matters. Avoiding alcohol, drugs, nicotine, and caffeine is good for us in the long run; when we are already in a weakened condition, avoiding these things can make us better able to fight the battle.

We need constantly to be making an assessment of what we can or cannot do at a particular stage. If we have overshot the mark, we need to pull back as gracefully as possible. If we are doing less than we can, we must endure the anxiety and discomfort of exerting ourselves a bit more.

Medications

Even when you follow your doctors orders carefully, you need to know exactly what medications and dosages you are taking—including over-the-counter drugs. Gather all your medications and put them on a table. Sort them out and list them on a piece of paper. Answer these questions.

- What is the drug for and what is it supposed to do?
- What are the side effects? Are they worth it?
- Will the drug react with other medications I'm taking?
- When does this prescription expire?
- Is this drug addicting?
- When is the best time to take this medication?

Take this list with you to your next doctor appointment and ask if you are getting the maximum from your medications.

Cracking Prescription Codes

Rx—prescription
Sig—label
AC—before meals
AD LIB—any time
BID—twice a day
PC—after meals
QD—every day
QH—every hour
QID—four times a day
QS—sufficient quantity
TID—three times a day
OS—left eye
OD—right eye

Having a *Physician's Desk Reference* available will help you identify and learn more about the medications you are using. The doctor will not always remember to forewarn you about possible side effects. Knowing some of these facts can ease your mind when strange symptoms pop up. If you have questions, your pharmacist is usually happy to provide information.

Nutrition

It has been proven time and again that a sensible diet can make you feel better even in spite of your chronic situation. Losing or gaining weight excessively and sporadically can cause flare-ups. If you need bed rest or use a wheelchair, you need to pay close attention to your weight. Learn what foods your body needs, and include these in your diet. Many situationers have food allergies and should see an allergist for treatment. He can run a series of tests and make changes in your diet. Check with your doctor about taking vitamin and mineral supplements. There are dozens of excellent books on nutrition that provide all the information you need. Your doctor may refer you to a nutritionist who can do a special evaluation of what you eat and what you need.

Exercise

Chronic situationers need to get as much physical exercise as possible. We need the physical stimulation, strengthening, and rejuvenation. Exercise strengthens muscles, burns calories, and conditions the heart. It also gives major psychological benefits and helps combat anxiety and depression. When we exercise, we are "in control," which is good for us mentally and emotionally. We decide how much to do and when to stop; just having that much control is a stress reliever. The physical tiredness caused by exercise makes us sleep better, thus improving our energy for the next day.

"Use it or lose it" is a true axiom. Whenever I'm hospitalized I ask for a bedframe with a trapeze that helps me move around in bed. This keeps me stronger so that when I go home I can again transfer from my bed to wheelchair on my own.

The body has an ample supply of natural tranquilizers on hand whenever they are needed. Exercise triggers the release of hormones into the blood stream. Taking a brisk walk not only lets off steam but releases endorphins and chemicals in the brain that can provide some pain relief.

All chronic situationers have different levels of disability. Before embarking on an exercise program, ask your doctor or physiotherapist for guidelines. The wrong kind of exercise or overexercise can harm more than help.

I think that exercise classes are the best way to go. You have someone to work with and a set time, which makes a program easier to stick with. These classes are provided by parks and recreation departments, the YMCA or YWCA, or other recreation centers. Some private health clubs and spas have developed classes for the disabled.

The easiest form of exercise is done in warm-water pools. The buoyancy of the water lessens impact and gives you a freedom of movement not possible out of water.

If you can no longer participate in some activities, choose others that are enjoyable to you. A paraplegic can't ride a conventional bicycle, but there are tricycles that can be propelled by the arms and shoulders. Regular sports may be in the past, but wheelchair sports are fun.

Physical therapy offers exercise. Massage to the legs and back increases circulation and prevents pressure sores. Having a physical therapist stretch out limbs can prevent muscle contractures.

Stop exercising when you experience nausea, chest pain, dizziness, breathlessness, fatigue, or other symptoms of distress. There are times in which you should not exercise—like when a body part is inflamed.

Rest

By *rest* I mean quiet relaxation. We cannot combat the stresses of illness without real rest. Rest when you're tired. Don't push activity until you're exhausted. It's so easy to overdo after a long period of not being able to do anything, but in the end we pay for not respecting our limitations.

What is a decent amount of rest for me may be too much or too little for someone else. Each of us has different rhythms that determine how much sleep we need. Too much sleep can make us tired and restless at bedtime but unable to sleep. Check with your doctor if you are having sleep disorders. Inability to sleep sometimes indicates depression; it always indicates that something is out of balance and needs to be addressed.

If you spend a lot of time in bed due to your condition, it's imperative that you have a bed that's good for you. It's also important that you have a place where you can totally relax. You may have to reconfigure the layout of the rooms in your house. You may have to buy a special bed or mattress. These are not luxury measures when you're in a chronic situation. Make the process enjoyable; employ the imaginations of your spouse, children, and friends as you create an attractive and restful physical environment for yourself and for them.

Attitude and Appearance

Take the time to dress well; take pride in yourself. "Like it or not, appearance is a very important part of your image and your self-esteem. You create an image that enhances your true self. You are one of a kind, as different from everyone else as a snowflake is different from every other snowflake. Let your uniqueness be the basis upon which you build the image you want to show the world." [3]

Attitudes *can* be changed. You don't have to like your disease or disability in order to accept it. And acceptance is not the same as pessimistic resignation.

Our lifestyle involves a number of different roles, e.g., spouse, parent, friend, student, churchgoer, employer, employee. Our self-image largely determines how others treat us. For example: A person with a spinal cord injury is faced with the hard facts that he is now different from what he was before his injury. He hates the change and may overgeneralize: " 'If I can't walk, I can't think, I can't be loved and I am really worthless.' Or he may oversimplify: 'I want nothing, I expect nothing, I don't care' to protect himself from the vulnerability of hoping and being disappointed again." [4]

For most people the mental aspects of a chronic situation become harder to overcome than the illness itself. Someone who has a positive attitude toward their situation has arrived there only with the hard work of self-control and positive thinking.

The world really does see us as we see ourselves. If someone with a problem feels embarrassed, the problem may not show, but the embarrassment will. Consequently others will feel embarrassed for him. On the other hand, if we are content and have respect for ourselves, the people we meet will respond to our mood. We must remember that we are first of all *persons,* not diseases or conditions.

> *No one can make you feel inferior without your consent.—Eleanor Roosevelt*

Practicing a positive attitude is difficult but necessary for everyone involved in a chronic situation. We need to be kind to ourselves. We must hug ourselves if we can't find anyone to hug us. We aren't cursed because of our situation; it is not our fault.

When we're unable to attend to our everyday functions, we are reminded that our very existence is part of God's plan and purpose. What we *are* is more important than what we can do.

When we accept ourselves, the anger, depression, and rejection will be lost in the tenderness, forgiveness, and love that comes when any person accepts who he is and where he is. In this acceptance there will be peace.

Establishing priorities is important for everyone, but a chronic situationer often has more limitations in time and energy. Notice where you waste time. Ask yourself where you spin your wheels. Prune out the deadwood from your life. Spend more time with positive people. Let go of people who drag you down.

We situationers also need time alone. Some questions we can ask ourselves:

- How do I really feel about my illness or accident?
- Have I really accepted my situation?
- How do I now see myself?
- How does this affect my relationships?
- What is the most important area of my life?
- What do I do that is right? What can I change for a better attitude?
- What do I fear the most? What can I do about it?
- What do I really enjoy in life? What has become a burden?
- How can I get on with the business of living?
- What are my feelings about death?

Take time out from tension by spending time alone in a peaceful place. Close your eyes for several minutes and breathe in fresh air. Take mini-vacations and go anywhere you fancy in your mind.

Find Someone Who Will Listen

When we are able to express our needs and concerns to others who understand, we are better able to overcome fears and frustrations. A chronically ill or disabled person needs people who will listen without judgment. Talking about problems doesn't always solve them, but it does reduce stress. And often a close friend or relative can look at our situation with new eyes and point out factors we have failed to see.

Sometimes our needs go beyond the scope of caring, listening friends and family members. Struggles can become too complex for people who do not have professional training as counselors. And sometimes our struggles involve the very people who would try to help us—such as our caregivers. Where do you turn when you are experiencing all sorts of conflicting emotions about your mother, who stays with you regularly, or your spouse?

If you feel that you need professional help, don't let embarrassment or guilt prevent you from getting it. A chronic situation has plenty of potential for creating big mental and emotional struggles that the average person cannot manage alone. Counseling options are numerous. You may need one-on-one counseling. If so, choose a counselor you can connect with. This might be a trained psychotherapist or a member of the clergy. Keep in mind the needs that you are addressing; this will make a difference in the kind of help you seek. We wouldn't let just anyone do surgery on our bodies; we must feel confident that our minds and emotions will get the best treatment also.

Joining a support group is another option, and it can help us interact with others in similar situations. New friendships can develop and a general network can form in these groups. It always helps us to know we are not alone. You can find support groups through local newspapers, hospitals, counseling centers, or universities. See appendix B for a listing of national support groups. Support groups are discussed in greater detail in chapter 7.

Learn Outward Motion

There are times when the best thing you can do is forget yourself and be completely interested in another person. If we don't learn to focus outwardly part of the time, we will merely become a manifestation of our illness or disability.

You don't have to be feeling well to invite people to your house. They don't expect glitzy treatment. You don't have to cook or clean. I cherish the many fast food lunches I've shared at my bedside with friends.

Church attendance and fellowship with other believers are key means of getting outside of ourselves. The very heart of the Good News is giving, serving, and loving others. Notice that none of the commandments to love others are contingent upon our lives being in good condition first. Jesus first said "Love one another" to a group of ordinary people whom he knew would have hardships in their lives. You won't be excused from Christian living because you are ill; your form of the Christian life will simply develop its own, unique angles.

Too much solitude becomes frustrating, anyway. You need to go where the action is! You have gifts to offer in your community and church. Your health will benefit as you get involved with the problems and adventures that are out there in the world. Even if you are homebound there is always something you can do. At times you certainly won't feel like doing anything. But I've found that after I've decided to get busy I can still enjoy activities.

> *To feel good about yourself do this—start giving. Give yourself to someone in some service that you do not need to give. Just let yourself flow out to people. This will make you feel awfully good about yourself.—Norman Vincent Peale*

What Is Your Purpose?

Chronic situationers need to have a purpose in life, just like everyone else. People who have "places to go and things to do" live longer. Many of us would not be alive now were it not for the purpose derived in fighting illness; there are times when that's all we have to go on. But there's a larger reason for us to be alive. Give attention to this question: What is my purpose in life? It's not a question this book or any other can answer for you; each person must take his or her own journey.

Along with a general goal in life, we need diversions and companionship. As long as we are able we should go to work, take the kids to the zoo, play cards with friends, and travel.

We derive a sense of purpose from the acts of service we perform for others. There are thousands of acts of human service that have emerged from the experiences of chronic situationers and their families. Hundreds of grants, funds, and volunteer programs have been set up to help others have a higher quality of life than those situationers who have gone before them. Most organizations for helping people with specific diseases or disabilities were created by people who had some connection to the disease—through a friend or family member. If these people had not gone after purposeful living, where would the research be now? The helping organizations? It all started somewhere.

Some people offer their bodies for scientific research; others offer specific organs for transplantation. Laura cherished her eyesight and made arrangements to have her eyes transplanted when she knew she was soon to die. Her doctor announced at her funeral services that the cornea transplant had been successful and that a young boy would now be able to see. The thought that Laura was able to provide something valuable was meaningful to her family. Acts of human service lift us beyond our circumstances— and they enrich the lives of others.

> *What we have done for ourselves alone dies with us. What we have done for others and the world remains and is immortal.—Albert Pine*

Rediscovering the God Who Loves Us

Somewhere along our journey we will enter the "dark night of the soul." It may be a sense of exhaustion, depression, or aloneness. There is a sense of separateness from God and an inability to cope. We wonder if God is really there. Everyone around us sleeps peacefully while we face our fears alone.

We must keep in mind that all these doubts and fears are not strange or abnormal in God's sight. To him it is part of the lifelong process that acquaints us with his grace. We look at ourselves and see a mere, short lifetime—one that may be cut shorter by our illness. Yet God sees us in the context of eternity and therefore he's not in a rush. He only wants us to learn how much we are loved by him. These dark nights of the soul are just one way of helping us settle down enough to listen and be aware of the God who is with us, the God who truly cares for us. He doesn't expect us to understand all at once; struggle is just part of the process. The best thing we can do sometimes is *give up* trying to make sense out of our situation. The best thing we can do is say, "God, help me. I'm clueless." When we get to that point, the morning is on its way—and God brings us to a hush, a stillness so that he may work an inner transformation.

I have come to sense God's nearness. We can talk to him about everything. When we come to our Father in prayer, we don't need to put on airs or masks. He knows us through and through and, as our Father, he loves it when we take the time to truly fellowship with him.

We can cry out as the psalmist did in Psalm 13:1: "How long, O LORD? Will you forget me forever?" He will listen to our cry and come alongside of us saying, "Do not be anxious about anything, but in everything, by prayer and petition, with thanksgiving, present your requests to God. And the peace of God, which transcends all understanding, will guard your hearts and your minds in Christ Jesus" (Philippians 4:6-7).

Don't forget praise and music. Singing praise songs can improve our moods and attitudes. We don't need to have musical talent. God loves the praise of his people and loves us the way we are. In a recent issue of *Christianity Today,* a married couple's ministry was highlighted. What do they do? They sing, read Scriptures, and pray at the bedsides of comatose patients. Not only do they see response on the faces of these people, but they have seen entire families changed through this simple ministry of song and Scripture.

Prayer can become a way of life, an approach to our chronic situation. When we ask others to pray for us we are mobilizing God's prayer warriors. Flooding the heavens with prayers is very powerful and can lead us to hope.

Encouragement along the Way

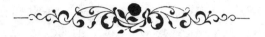

*L*ord, transform my suffering into growth, my tears into prayer, my discouragement into faith, my fears into trust, my expectations into hopes, my anger into closeness, my bitterness into acceptance, my guilt into reconciliation, my loneliness into contemplation, my silence into peace, my deaths into resurrection. Amen.

9

Coping as a Family

Dear friends, let us love one another, for love comes from God. Everyone who loves has been born of God and knows God. Whoever does not love does not know God, because God is love.—1 John 4:7-8

The diagnosis and treatment of a chronic disease or disability can deliver unexpected blows to a family's sense of security, their plans and dreams.

There are more than thirty-five million disabled individuals in this country. Sixty million more are seriously ill. Add to that figure the millions of family members who are greatly affected, and you have an astounding figure. These families are on a roller coaster along with their ill family members. A chronic situation, even if it is not immediately life-threatening, imposes a great number of hardships on a family. Their lives have been permanently changed.

Spinal cord injuries can have a catastrophic impact on a person's emotional status—an impact that extends to the families of the injured as well.—Donald S. Pierce and Vernon H. Nickel[1]

Who Should Be Told—And How Much Should They Be Told?

Each person involved in a chronic situation needs to be told the truth. By involving your loved ones, it gives them the opportunity to offer their support. Educating family members about your situation helps them to be involved intelligently. Some might not be able to handle this information; they might slip away, but others will be willing to help. Chronic situationers should not have to bear the situation alone. And, eventually, the entire family must face the situation.

Children should not be kept in the dark. They can sense when something is amiss, and they tend to imagine a situation worse than it really is when left on their own. Our children were preschoolers when my disease surfaced. We couldn't protect them from the truth. We tried to make it part of our lives. (More about this later in the chapter.)

How much should be told? This is a difficult question and the "right" answer depends on the medical condition involved, the stage you are at presently, and the makeup of your family. Some people can make a matter worse through unnecessary worry or hysteria; telling them every detail as the condition unfolds may not be a good idea. Others feel the need to know everything so that they can be with you through it and can pray specifically.

People with unseen conditions are often misunderstood. Others may slap you on the back and say, "You're looking great!" when in fact you're feeling lousy. People don't mean to hurt you. That might be an appropriate time to tell your family members about your health or injury and accompanying problems. It is up to you to teach them about your condition and help them know the truth about how you feel at times.

When people see you out in public they assume you're feeling quite well. What most do not know is how you rested all morning to be able to attend a luncheon and immediately when you get home you will need to rest again.

Ironically, the person who is ill must make judgment calls on how to aid others in helping him or her. This involves decisions about whom to tell what. And how an ill person handles the situation is automatically a living example to others.

Georgia and Bud Photopulos talk about how audiences were astounded when they first saw Georgia because she didn't look like she had survived two mastectomies and undergone extensive radiation and chemotherapy. The reason for the surprise was "she never permitted herself to give in to her illness, to its side effects on either her health or her appearance."[2] She wore makeup and a wig.

"Unfortunately people expect to see you bleeding and bandaged, on crutches or in a wheelchair. . . . Her healthy appearance enabled her to convey the positive side of cancer—the chance for cure if caught early enough and the expectation of resuming a productive life after treatment. . . . She was able to reach patients and nonpatients, health care professionals, clergy, researchers and fund-raisers."[3] She gave a message of hope. Chronic situationers must learn how to be honest, yet positive.

You'll notice that whenever a chronic situation comes into a family, everyone becomes a medical expert. For example, Aunt Sally knows of a person who had a similar disease and goes on to tell you about that person's treatment and how it helped. These comments should be handled in a positive way—if possible. One woman strongly suggested to me that if I would sit naked on a stool with a towel over my head and pour cold water down my front, I would be healed. She showed me a diagram in a book that was published in 1909. I gently and calmly told her thanks for thinking of me. I asked her to continue to pray for me and my family. At a time in your life when you may need extra support from extended family, you may be called upon to show extra understanding for them.

I wrote my family a letter explaining that I had Acute Intermittent Porphyria and gave some honest and basic information about my disease. Each family member dealt with it in his or her own way. Both my brother and sister expressed anger, but once that had passed they were able to provide support and love.

Grieving As a Family

> *Strength of character may be acquired at work, but beauty of character is learned at home. There the affections are trained. There the gentle life reaches us, the true heaven life. In one word, the family circle is the supreme conductor of Christianity.*—Henry Drummond

Relatives go through the same stages of grief the patient experiences. And no one goes through them in quite the same way as anyone else.

When a patient is diagnosed, that family and individual often deny the existence of a serious condition. *Denial* can enable the individual and his family to get through an early adjustment phase. Absorbing the diagnosis takes time and energy, but soon everyone involved must face the facts. Each family member needs to sort out the feelings of death and fear in his or her good time.

Anger too can be healthy. It can motivate a person to yell, "I'm so angry. I'm going to show everyone that they are wrong. I'm going to live in spite of everyone's predictions."

Family members also can find the extra energy from anger that they need to fight the situation this disease or injury has brought. It's important, though, that "anger energy" be channeled properly; this is not the time to be sparring with one another. If the family can come together and recognize that they have a common enemy—this situation—and agree not to "beat up" on one another, some real progress can be made. As much as we don't want to hurt one another, it's too easy to allow our anger to spill out on the people we love most.

Once reality hits, anger turns inward and causes *depression*. The situationer has this treatment today and next week there will be more therapy, tests, and procedures. Suddenly the whole family feels that they have no control of their lives. An otherwise active, productive family member has become ill or injured and needs much assistance. That can feel like an overwhelming burden to the family, no matter how much love exists.

> *In times of intense physical pain, confusion, and doubt, one must simply decide and do, decide and do—and laugh a bit amidst the consequences.*
> *—Unknown*

Stresses on the Family

You should never underestimate the importance of family when living in a chronic situation. Family members, as well as the patient, should be part of the treatment team. "Family members must deal with life both inside and outside the hospital. You must try to find the energy and ability to be supportive of the patient, maintain other family commitments, and carry out the business of the day-to-day activities. The patient knows that there is a hospital staff available 24 hours a day to meet his physical and emotional needs, but who is available to lend support to the family?"[4]

In a chronic situation much time is spent with repeated doctor appointments, hospitalizations, treatments, examinations, tests, x-rays, and physical therapy. Often the treatments cause pain and anxiety. Sometimes the patient has used all his resources just to cope. There is no extra energy to share with the family. Chronic situations are emotionally and physically draining for families.

Going to doctor appointments can take three to four hours. If you are the spouse of the ill person, you may have to take time off from work. You might need child care. All kinds of questions occur and add to the stress:

- Who will watch the kids?
- Will the children worry that I'm not coming back?
- What if this turns into another hospital stay?
- Can they get along without me at work?

> *"Life must go on, I forget just why," but the routine of meals is itself part of life and part of the mechanism of coping.—Edna St. Vincent Millay*

Repeated hospitalizations can take their toll on a family; that prospect is like a strong undercurrent, threatening to pull all of you out to sea. Sometimes for a short while a family can forget about the chronic situation, but the reality of it always hovers.

It is stressful for loved ones to sit by and watch their family member decline and live in pain. We can't hide our chronic condition from our loved ones. The whole extended family hurts. Any loss we have is also a loss to each family member.

For the Family Member Who Wants to Help

Keep in mind that the ill person in your family already feels like a burden—financially, physically, emotionally, and spiritually. This sometimes leads to frustration and hopelessness. The ill member will withdraw from the rest of you at times. He or she will be in physical discomfort or downright pain. Sometimes a chronically ill person is agitated and can't keep still; he or she moves constantly, has difficulty getting rest or sleep, and is unable to slow down racing thoughts.

How do you help a person with such a wide and serious fluctuation of needs? The most obvious trait you need to develop is flexibility—the ability to stay away or push closer, to just sit and listen without judgment or comment, or to have an abundance of hopeful and encouraging (yet honest and realistic!) things to say when he or she falls into sad silence and needs to hear you.

There are some very practical ways of helping worth listing here:

Learn to be a good listener.

Be present—for doctor and treatment appointments, when the person is having surgery and afterwards, to help sort out information and instructions the surgeon and other doctors may have.

Express encouragement. Point out good responses to treatment. Allow the person to do as much for himself as possible and remind him of what he is *able* to do.

Avoid pity. Especially avoid false cheer—"Everything will be all right. Cheer up." Everything will *not* be all right. This

143

kind of hiding from the truth can be devastating to a situationer.

Educate yourself about the loved one's condition, so that you have a fuller understanding of what she's going through.

Treat your family member as an adult. The patient appreciates your concerns, but telling the patient to "go lie down—you look tired" is demeaning. The patient has given up so much of her independence already; she doesn't need excessive instructions on taking care of herself.

Extend regular invitations to get your family member out of the house. If you usually go out for special occasions, try to keep the routine going. It's okay to try a little coaching if your invitation is declined, but don't push too hard.

Maintain an attitude of hope. To some extent, this means doing your best to carry on the activities you have always shared. It also means reaching together for support and help. One of the best ways of doing this is to pray together.

> *Those dear to us should never be denied the knowledge of how deeply they have touched our lives.—Marcia Van't Land*

Family Counseling

We cope with a chronic illness or disability much as we cope with other problems that confront us. We need to be realistic but also optimistic.

In the cases of accident or traumatic injury there is often a need "to have all family members visit the occupational and physical therapy sessions to observe the rehabilitation program in action. By doing so, they become more realistic about the abilities of the patient and at the same time better understand some of the adjustment problems facing the patient."[5]

> *As time passes, you'll find that those precious ones who are able to go the distance with you become rare treasures and that the real wealth of this life is to be found in those relationships.*
> *—Kathleen Lewis*

Often the patient will make progress in accepting the injury, but when he comes home one of his family members may say, "You just keep trying, and you will walk" or, "We are praying for you, and we know that God will not let you down." They undo the work of the occupational and physical therapists because of their own feelings of helplessness. *Acceptance* is a process they have not dealt with (it is also the final stage of grief). Family members need an opportunity to discuss their own feelings regarding the total picture. Often they have guilt feelings, almost always unfounded, associated with the event that caused the injury. Some families can discuss the situation, but others can't and need outside help.

Large hospitals have programs for family and friends. When my friend's husband had bypass surgery, they were required to attend classes informing them how to eat healthily and exercise.

Psychological counseling in the form of group therapy with other families can also be helpful. Support groups that share common fears and concerns with others who are experiencing essentially the same thing offer a unique kind of support and encouragement.

Other times individual counseling for a family member is needed. It's not always possible to work through the range of emotions on our own. Remember that the illness or disability is a *family* problem; no one goes unaffected, and no one should feel ashamed about needing help in coping.

Financial Obligations

It takes a lot of money to fight a chronic situation. Many people do not understand this, especially if they haven't been in a long-term situation or responsible for someone's long-term care. Insurance doesn't cover everything. There are a lot of expenses related to medical care that most people don't think about—parking fees, travel expenses, telephone calls, hotel rooms, babysitters, maintenance on medical equipment, special supplies, medications, physical therapy, personal care attendants, vehicle maintenance (chair lifts and wheelchair repairs), and insurance deductibles. Most insurance companies cover the cost of the first wheelchair but pay nothing when a few years later you need a new one.

No insurance company likes to insure a chronic situationer. They lose money on us. Most of us pay high insurance premiums to cover the cost of basic coverage. We shudder to even think about changing insurance companies because they would place a waiver on us. In some cases people have even been dropped from coverage once they developed serious illness or disability.

Loving costs a lot, but not loving always costs more.—Helen Macinness

Not only are insurance premiums high, but a chronic situationer is often unable to hold down a job and contribute to the family income. Some don't have the energy to strategize the use of money—such as shopping around for the best prices on normal household goods.

The amount of paperwork involved in submitting bills to the insurance company is staggering. Tom has a large filing box full of insurance papers. He spends hours keeping all our medical bills updated.

My disease affects my gums and teeth, so we have added dental bills that insurance doesn't cover.

There are no easy answers to these financial dilemmas. Situationers walk a fine line between letting their needs be known to others and managing as well as they can without additional help. Financial planning is a good idea, but it only takes a relapse or some new treatment to dismantle the most carefully laid plans; a chronic illness or disability brings *unpredictability* into the financial picture.

Not only is it difficult to accept that you have permanent financial limitations, it's a challenge to convey to your children that money really is not the measure of our worth. They will learn by *your* example and *your* attitude that, if you never own a new car or move to a nicer house or go on a vacation cruise, life will still be okay. More than ever, it becomes necessary to build family traditions and generate family activities that make home truly *home*, regardless of economic status.

These kinds of issues are faced daily by families involved in a chronic situation. There are many sacrifices by all involved. Our family relationships need to be based on love and a willingness to share all problems together. Families pulling together in spite of difficulties can present the best Christian witness to all those who come in touch with the family.

The Children

Serious illness or accident can be traumatic for children, since they are so vulnerable. They may hear relatives whispering or snatches of phone conversations. They sense something is wrong and become afraid and insecure. Perhaps the adult from whom the children get emotional support is unable to nurture them at times.

However, if a child grows up with a parent who is a situationer, he or she accepts the situation as normal. Until our children were five or six, they assumed everyone's mom went to the hospital as often as I did. They accepted my wheelchair as normal, too. One day they asked me, "Why can't you walk like Katie's mom?" We knew then that our children needed more explanation about my disease and the changes it was making in our lives.

> *Merely coping with problems and tragedies is not enough. We need to go beyond any trust by using it for growth and development.—Unknown*

We had a family meeting. We were honest and told them exactly what was happening with my disease. We weren't explicit with all the details but answered their questions. Including too much detail can be overwhelming for children. We told them we loved them very much and that we were a family who would hang in there together.

During this time of adjustment, children may become preoccupied with death. This is normal, and we will address this topic in a later chapter.

Teenagers are often concerned about fitting in with their peer group and may not want to tell their friends about your chronic condition. They may react in anger or they may try to ignore it. Don't force them to talk. They will in their own time express the fears and questions they have. Don't be disappointed if they express themselves to someone besides you. Be grateful for teachers, church members, and other adult friends who will help your children maintain their equilibrium. It is healthy for them to learn what resources they have outside the family. Keep in mind, though, that *they still need you.* They need to hear you say, "I love you" or, "How about a hug?" Showing your appreciation for the household responsibilities they have had to assume can be a great way of relating to them.

Older teens and adult children may be more mature and independent, but they need to be involved in the situation. Their questions will be more detailed and won't be as easy to answer. They often benefit from reading literature about your situation and then discussing it with you later. You may not have answers to all their questions, but if you stress learning about it together, it will ease their minds.

Helping Your Children Deal with a Chronic Situation

Listen to them and answer their questions.

Try to keep your home life as normal as possible.
Children need routine in their lives.

Reevaluate priorities often. Relax cleaning standards and spend your good time with the family, not in frantically trying to keep a clean house and yard.

Make your children feel that your situation is a family affair and that you'll face it together. Make it a challenge and an adventure.

Be consistent with discipline. Kids need lots of love, and their need for structure and boundaries doesn't disappear just because you are ill. When children are asked to play quietly, provide materials that will keep them interested and occupied.

If a lengthy, distant hospitalization occurs, stay in touch by telephone and send presents or postcards. When hospitalized locally, arrange times for the children to visit you. Even when our children were very young, my doctor would always write on my chart that it was permissible for them to visit. This helped my morale and theirs. Sometimes it told me that I wasn't well enough to come home to all their energy. It is important to prepare for the visit. Explain that mom will be in bed wearing a hospital gown. She will have a needle in her arm to get medicine in her body so she can get better.

Have regular family devotions and pray together. If the children see and hear your trust in the Lord, they will feel more secure.

Enjoy each day as a gift and appreciate your time with your children.

Lessons Learned As a Family

1. Budget your time and energy. Continually ask yourself what is more important. Should you go to a meeting or use your energy to shop for a banquet dress for your daughter? What is going to be important ten years from now?

2. Children raised with a chronic situation are often more tolerant, aware, and sensitive to the limitations of others. If the parents accept the situation, then the children will feel the same.

3. The financial budget can be quite limited, but you can enjoy cheaper activities and be together.

4. Try to take the focus off the chronic situation. It is healthy for family members to have outside interests and goals.

5. Slow down. " We can affirm the value of life, of close relationships, of meaningful dreams that God has embedded in our hearts."[6]

6. Allow other adults to be parents to your children at times. The extra

attention is important.
7. Visitors come to see you and not to inspect your house. Being relaxed no matter what the situation is will encourage family and friends to visit again.
8. If you can afford outside help, do so. The family has enough stress—let someone else keep up the house and yard.
9. Focus on the things you are able to do and not on the things you can no longer enjoy.

Making Memories

Whether we admit it or not, each day we are making memories. Many of our family's memories center around how we coped with my disease.

One day when Tom and the kids were visiting me in the hospital, our four-year-old was curious about the emergency cord in the bathroom. She pulled it and instantly the room was crowded with nurses wondering what the emergency was. They opened the door and there she sat with a sheepish grin on her face.

Many times the walls of my "Jesus room" (what the nurses called my hospital room) were adorned with paintings and drawings of our children and their friends.

Special occasions needed to be celebrated in my hospital room. One night we turned off my oxygen before we lit the candles on birthday cupcakes baked by a friend for one of the children's birthdays.

Our children always visit me briefly when I'm in Intensive Care. It is always difficult and they always cry but we can't deny my illness. We must remember that even painful experiences, in a loving context, build strength in our children for the hard times they are bound to face throughout their lives. These kinds of memories will remind them that they have survived hardship in the past and will continue to survive and live with meaning and purpose.

Sometimes our children would ask me, "Mom, do you wish you had a different body?" I reply, "Yes, I surely do, but this is the way things are. I can't play soccer and run with you, but we can do all sorts of other things together, can't we?" They would sense when my pain was unbearable and would lovingly rub my back or just snuggle in our bed and talk. Then I would no longer feel like a useless blob scrunched up in bed.

When I'm in my electric wheelchair they ride their bikes in circles around me. What fun we have doing pop-a-wheelies, flying up and down the ramps.

Studies have shown that attitudes toward a chronic situation and how we deal with it are closely tied to the positive or negative feelings we sense from our families. Professionals, family, and friends can enable the individual to deal with the chronic situation in a positive way. If the family encourages the patient with hope and love, the patient adjusts in a positive manner.

Your home can be a refuge from the bruises and bumps of everyday life. "With enough time and enough communication, people can incorporate into their relationship the new norms and expectations brought on by a chronic situation."[7]

We have God's promise: "God is faithful: he will not let you be tempted beyond what you can bear. But when you are tempted, he will also provide a way out so that you can stand up under it" (1 Corinthians 10:13).

Encouragement along the Way

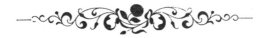

Still She Smiles

There she goes down the road
   in her old black wheelchair.
Watching children run and play,
   something she will never do again.
   Still she smiles.
Why does she keep on going through
   her pain and agony?
She keeps on going for her children
   and her husband.
   Still she smiles.
When she goes into the hospital
   she is very sad indeed.
She is weak and tired with tubes
   and IVs in her body.
   Still she smiles.
She has had her disease
   for twelve years.
Yet, her friends show her
   love and comfort.
   Still she smiles.
Even though she wants to jump up and run
   from all her sorrows
   she cannot go.
I don't want my mom's life to end.
   Still she smiles.

When will the road ever end?
I hope it's a long road.
  for I don't want her life
  to end.
  Still she smiles.
—Ruth Van't Land
March 1992
age twelve

10

Especially for Caregivers

Blessed are the merciful, for they will be shown mercy.—Matthew 5:7

A few years ago the word 'caregiver' was not a common one. Today that word describes several million unpaid friends or family members caring for relatives who are ill, have disabilities or are elderly."[1]

Many people who need assistance do not need to be institutionalized, and there are a variety of family members providing basic care. The primary caregiver can be a spouse, parent, other relatives, or friends. Being the primary caregiver may not be your choice but the patient needs help; because of your relationship to him or her the task falls on you.

Major illness constantly tests the strength of a marriage.—Unknown

In their book, *Of Tears and Triumphs,* Bud and Georgia Photopulos say, "When illness comes, it disrupts your life, demands huge chunks of time and energy, postpones your plans, reroutes your course, and frequently depletes your savings. It penetrates a family's life fabric as it invades the body, thrusting everyone onto an emotional battleground where tears and heartbreak are confronted daily."[2]

In Sickness and In Health

Chronic situations have impact on all relationships, but the relationship between husband and wife is most affected. Seventy-five percent of marriages end in divorce when one spouse has a life-threatening illness or becomes disabled in some way. Catastrophic illnesses and accidents have broken more homes than earthquakes and floods. The Red Cross and government agencies come around with assistance after natural disasters, but nobody bails you out of huge unpayable hospital and doctor bills. No one rescues an overtired caregiver. No one can take away a chronic situation.

The strain on a marriage is especially great when the wife is affected. In general, women are able to adjust and accommodate to the needs of becoming a caregiver. It is more difficult for a man to assume the responsibility of caring for an ill or injured wife. He may respond by working harder at his career. He wants to be a better provider but the affected wife wants him to spend more time with her. And so the merry-go-round begins and never ends.

> *X-rays are like a marriage. Your chances of hiding anything are poor.—Unknown*

Most of us have had experience as a caregiver for a short time. A broken bone or case of the flu are short-lived circumstances we can deal with quite well. Often a chronic situation means that an adult may not be able to care for himself completely. That fact alone is stressful. Being dependent on your spouse can cause a rift between the caregiver and the patient.

A healthy marriage is a partnership. After the courtship you settle in and work out a balance of responsibilities and roles. When a chronic situation occurs, the balance changes. It permanently changes. It is unplanned and uninvited. It permeates every facet of your lives together. Hearing the news that you have diabetes, MS, cancer, or a spinal cord injury can throw everyone involved into a tailspin.

We need to learn to respond to the crises that occur repeatedly. Emotions like guilt, fear, anger, depression, and resentment need to be worked through by both spouses. While a chronic illness can test you beyond what you thought possible, it can also reveal to you the strength you never dreamed you had. This situation can tear a relationship apart—but it can also stimulate a depth of love unknown in better times. As miracles—small and large—occur in your spirit, emotions, and body, both patient and caregiver are the recipients. As frightening as the divorce statistics are, this time, more than ever, is a time for committing yourselves to love and possibility thinking.

It's not uncommon for one of the spouses to withdraw during serious illness or injury. One man related tearfully, "My wife became seriously ill several months ago and our relationship has deteriorated to such an extent that I almost hate to go home. Our marriage has been happy and our relationship the best, but now I can't seem to do anything right and I'm at my wit's end."

The highs and lows, the decisions regarding care, and the emotional impact of caring for a family can overwhelm the well spouse. He is not excused from performing his normal duties and responsibilities as readily as the ill spouse. It may be impossible for him to concentrate on his work. He doesn't know whether he should neglect his work. He is afraid to ask for time off because his work is providing the medical insurance needed for his wife's illness. Financial concerns put an added burden on both spouses. The wife feels guilty that so much money goes into medically related bills.

The well spouse shares the burden of a chronic situation but often doesn't have the support system of the affected spouse. People don't visit him or bring him presents. The ill spouse often expresses anger, self-pity, and fear to the well spouse; then the well spouse feels guilty that he *is* well and becomes afraid of any negative feelings he may have. He mourns the lost marriage and lost family. The marriage becomes a pressure cooker of emotions ready to explode.

Tom and I have gone through the following stages over fifty times:

1. I have a few good weeks or months and gradually take on more responsibilities with our family and home.
2. I spend days in bed frantically trying to stay out of the hospital.
3. Tom finally brings me to the hospital and he and kids worry that I might die.
4. I return home and as I feel better I assume a more active role.
5. Tom and I have an argument. It always centers around the fact that Tom had all the responsibility for running our home. Even though he's glad that I'm improving he still considers me impinging on his domain.

On October 29, 1985, Tom wrote me the following note:

I'm very sorry for how I treated you yesterday. Please forgive me—as I know you will!

Things are not going well at work: I'm worried about our finances and housing situation; I get nothing done besides work and getting the kids to their stuff; I'm haunted by the prospect of losing you; I'm overwhelmed by all there is to do and pay for—especially for the kids.

But all of this is no excuse for mistreating you, and I will try not to do it again.

I love you and need you very much.

Ways to keep a relationship strong

The timing of the chronic situation has an effect on the coping skills of the marriage. If the situation was known and understood before the relationship began, the marriage will be stronger. The well spouse is least likely to say, "I want out. I want a wife who can ski and play sports. I can't handle this."

Generally, one would think that, the longer the marriage, the greater its strength. That isn't always true. Many relationships are fragile, and when a chronic situation is added the bond may break. *A chronic situation exposes a relationship for what it is.* Individual commitment is what counts. When a couple accepts these challenges, they can support one another and restore the balance that was there before.

> *We must resemble each other a little in order to understand each other, but we must be a little different to love each other.—Paul Geraldy*

How do we keep a relationship strong in the midst of the chronic illness storm? Each husband and wife must work out their own situation, but there are some principles that cut across individual differences.

Communicate. Put all the physical ailments aside and listen to one another from the heart. Work through difficult times *together.* Communication means talking about the chronic situation and how it has affected your relationship. Both partners can be angry at the disease or disability and express their negative emotions together without becoming personal. It takes a lot of commitment, but a married couple needs to regard the chronic situation as *our* disease or injury.

The two of you may not adjust to the chronic situation at the same time. You may be in the acceptance phase of grief while your partner is still in denial or depression. You need to allow room for your spouse to work through each phase.

> *If we are to make a mature adjustment to life, we must be able to give and receive love.—Unknown*

Make sure your marriage is not totally disease-focused. It is important for both spouses to have other interests and concerns. When she is social, she should be able to go out with her friends. If he is content watching a ballgame, he should enjoy that. Each one is happy that the other is having a good time. Selfish love is when she drags him out or he keeps her home.

Use as much outside help for gardening, babysitting, housecleaning, transportation, and whatever else can be done by hired help or by friends and family. This helps the well spouse have some free time for activities other than household chores.

Be flexible in roles. A couple that adheres to a strict definition of male and female roles will have to confront these values when a chronic situation occurs. Who does what and when is going to change.

When I first became ill, Tom assumed many of my roles out of necessity. When a friend of ours had a disabling accident, the wife needed to go to work full-time.

The ill spouse needs to encourage and appreciate what the well spouse does for the family. Plenty of thank yous and praise will help keep the well spouse motivated in his or her caregiver role.

It bothered me to see Tom under so much stress. I would try my hardest to relieve him of child care and household chores. In some ways I protected Tom and the kids from seeing all of my pain. I didn't want to be more of a burden than I already was. This protection was motivated by my love for them. If I fell apart, the whole family went with me.

> *If you let it, your chronic illness will change the orientation of your relationship away from nurturing each other and towards nurturing it. Your illness can become the focus of your relationship, making an awkward triangle: you, your spouse, and it.—Sefra Kobrin Pitzele*

Get professional help if needed. If you and your spouse have a difficult time communicating, professional marriage counseling might be good for you—it might become absolutely necessary. Bouncing ideas and attitudes off an objective, trained person can clear up misunderstandings that you are unaware of.

Be aware of how self-image changes. Over the years a person develops an image in her mind about her body. She may not be completely satisfied with that image but she is comfortable with it. If a disease or accident has changed your appearance, you wonder if your husband still finds you attractive, or if he is ashamed of how you look. If he says that it doesn't matter to him or he loves you just the same, you wonder if he's only saying that not to hurt your feelings.

> *Life is more than our bodies. The things that make us truly human and truly divine are not physical qualities.—R. Scott Sullender*

When a person is thirty pounds heavier because of medication or treatments, she may believe that she is no longer attractive, and this can affect the sexuality in the marriage.

Betsy Burnham, in her book *When Your Friend Is Dying,* asked her husband how he felt about her—with graying, thinning hair and a huge scar striping her abdomen. Her husband writes, "I realized that she wanted honesty—not flattery—and she wanted assurance. . . . Honey, I like you better with hair and without a scar—I admit that. But I love you just the same."

Betsy pursued it further. "Since I've been sick I know it has been tough for you—sexually I mean. I guess your physical needs aren't really being fulfilled, are they?"[3]

Monty, her husband, again responded honestly and openly, "No, my physical needs haven't been met. But you know there's more to our marriage than our physical relationship."

"What about sex?" is not the most important question anymore. The well spouse needs to find ways to communicate to his ill wife that he still finds her attractive in spite of her physical differentness.

On the other hand, "Patients should not be harsh with their loved ones if they temporarily pull away. If they were loving and attentive before diagnosis and treatment, they probably won't change, but they may need time to deal with their own fears and anxieties before they can be supportive.

"Expect that the spouse will not have identical feelings: every person reacts differently under stress. But it is important that you share how the experience affects each of you."[4]

Your husband may be aware of your fatigue, pain, and health concerns. A decrease in sexual attraction doesn't necessarily mean a decrease in love. Sexual intimacy might take a lot of creativity and imagination. Being able to hold one another can be fulfilling. A kiss or a pat on the back brings you closer than a thousand words. Countless times I'd lay my head on Tom's chest as he rubbed my back. We would lie there in the dark wondering how long we'd be able to enjoy this closeness. In the long run, it is love, caring, and concern, rather than sexual activity, that keeps a relationship alive.

If a couple is having sexual problems, this too can be discussed with a counselor. Don't be afraid to talk to your medical doctor or specialist; they see sexual difficulties in the context of the condition and know better than anyone that these problems are part of the package and not a reflection of the quality of your marriage.

Needs of the Caregiver

1. The employer of the caregiver needs to be apprised of the medical condition of the patient. Caregivers may need time off to take the patient to doctor appointments, therapy, or for general care at home when things are particularly bad or help cannot be found. An understanding employer can make it easier for the caregiver.
2. If the patient is bedridden, the caregiver needs part-time nursing assistance accordingly. The caregiver may need some respite help if family and friends cannot help out.
3. The caregiver needs positive support from family and friends. He needs someone to listen to his feelings and hurts. A pat on the back or saying, "I admire you for hanging in there" gives a lift to tired shoulders and spirit.
4. Live and face one day at a time. Dwelling on the future and what it may hold often borrows trouble and stress. Try to accept your present situation as a meaningful part of life.

5. Limits need to be set. There are things that we think are necessary but really aren't. Let go of some of these things and relax some standards.

6. Take care of yourself. Eat right, exercise, and save time for relaxation away from caregiver responsibilities.

7. Deal directly and cope with emotions such as loneliness, guilt and anger. Keep hope alive.

8. Join a caregiver's support group or go for one-on-one counseling. People involved in these groups can help you work through problems and cope with your situation. Call Community Care Resources: 612/642-4060 to receive an updated list of groups in your area.

9. Use services that are available in your area. *Take Care* is a guide for caregivers on how to improve their self-care. It is available by sending $2.50 to:
   Amherst H. Wilder Foundation
   Take Care!
   919 Lafond Ave.
   St. Paul, MN 55104

What helps the most when caregiving makes you tired or down?

I posed this question to forty-five caregivers. Below are some of their answers:

- "I find time alone, not having to deal with it for a day or so, to be most helpful to me when I need a recharge."
- "We go out to family and friends, and we do a lot of praying. I work out of the home two days a week and that helps me gain perspective."
- "Hearing a please or thank you is so important. At times I feel I'm only here to work, work, work because when a person has a chronic disease they focus on themselves easily."
- "Talking to a friend helps me."
- "The best help is my morning quiet time with my God. I can pour out all my fears and anxieties, and he not only understands, but he can change things. He gives me peace."
- "I find that if I can keep very busy I'm best off. At times it does help to talk to someone about my frustration. Just thinking out loud relieves some of the stress."
- "My Bible study group supports me in prayer."
- "I know God gave us to each other and we have never doubted our love. That helps a lot. I get tired sometimes but it helps that I know my husband is doing what he can—not just giving up."

Personal Care Attendants

Many disabled or ill persons are totally independent. Others can manage with the help of family and friends. But there are times when family help gets tired or needs a rest. They need time off for pursuing their own interests. Hiring either a full-time or part-time personal care attendant to assist with dressing, bathing, and other personal cares of daily living can be the answer.

For more information on personal care attendants, send for the book:

Home Health Aides: Manage the People Who Help You
by Al De Graff
Accent Special Publications
Box 700
Bloomington, IL 61702

In-Home Health Care

In some cases, patients need ongoing health and medical care after they leave the hospital. To keep the rising costs of hospitalization down, many families turn to In-Home Health Care.

The physician usually orders home care and the social worker or discharge planner contacts the Home Health agency and discusses the services you may need.

Visiting Nurses Association or Home Health Care offers RNs to monitor your blood pressure and pulse. They will give injections, dispense medications, change catheters and bandages.

The VNA also provides home aides who will help with bathing, dressing, and meal preparations.

Physical therapy, speech therapy, and occupational therapy services are also offered. Usually a social worker is affiliated with the Home Health Agency and can help coordinate these services. The social worker can offer individual or

169

family counseling to help assure that the transition back home goes as smoothly as possible.

Many communities provide "Meals on Wheels" programs that provide hot or cold meals that adhere to the diet restrictions of the individual patient. These meals are delivered directly to the home for a small fee.

The Home Health services are covered by Medicaid and Medicare, if a physician orders them. An RN must participate in the in-home care plan for you to get Medicare and Medicaid coverage. That is also true for most insurance coverage.

A helpful book on providing home care is:

> *Home Care: An Alternative to the Nursing Home*
> by Florine Du Fresne
> The Brethren Press
> Elgin, IL 60120

More than seven million Americans care for an older, often mentally impaired, adult in their homes. Eventually they may need outside help. To learn more about taking care of an older dependent, both at home and elsewhere, write:

> Family Survival Project
> 425 Bush St., Ste. 500
> San Francisco, CA 94108
> (Fact sheets "Caregiving" and "Placement Options" free with $1.00 check for postage and handling.)

> Alzheimer's Association
> P.O. Box 567HC
> Chicago, IL 60680-5675
> (Booklet "Steps to Finding Home Care" is $1.50 check or money order.)

Nursing Homes

When caregiving in the home is no longer an option, the patient and family members must come to terms with the idea of a nursing home. Initially, a patient and family may be saddened or afraid when the physician recommends a nursing home placement. A nursing home does not necessarily have to be a place where the patient goes to die. They often feel better when they learn about the quality of care most nursing homes offer.

Nursing homes offer three levels of care: skilled (infirmary), intermediate (group home), and extended care facilities (cottages or apartments).

Research is a must when considering a nursing home. Find out the following:

- Is the home licensed? Ask. If the answer is yes, ask to see the license.
- Does the administrator have a current state license? Again, ask to see it.
- Is the nursing home Medicare and Medicaid approved?
- What other insurance plans are accepted?
- Are there additional charges for personal laundry? Does therapy cost extra, and if so, how much?
- Are residents allowed to furnish their rooms with their own furniture? Can residents have their own radios or televisions?
- Can a husband and wife share the same room?
- Are residents permitted to smoke in their rooms? If so, are they supervised? What about alcoholic beverages?
- Are there restrictions on making or receiving phone calls?

- What are the visiting hours?
- Where is the residents' money kept? Are there provisions for personal banking services?
- When was the last state or local inspection, and what were the results?
- How often are fire drills held for staff and residents?
- What types of recreational activities are available to residents? Don't hesitate to ask to see the schedule of activities.
- How are residents' medical needs met? Does the nursing home have an arrangement with a nearby hospital to handle emergencies?
- Are special diets available for those who need them? Is there a professional dietitian on the staff who is available as a consultant?[5]

Caregivers perform a higher service because they not only provide care but they work to serve God. Joni Eareckson Tada reminds us that "the Lord Jesus will neither overlook nor forget the task you (caregivers) perform in His name. Nor will he fail to reward you."[6]

Encouragement along the Way

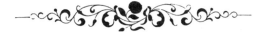

*S*piritual Lifts from Caregivers

- "I try to focus on the unchanging aspects of God's character—the only thing we can trust. If God allowed us to see around the corner, we wouldn't go. He knows what we need and will supply it if we come and ask."

- "One of my personal struggles is the role of God in illness. The older more traditional view of a sovereign God who sends adversity does not sit well with me anymore. My view of God's sovereignty has changed. He is much more a friend who is with us in our struggles in this broken world than a God who sends illnesses and accidents and then, as it were, sees how we react to it. I find Philip Yancey's books to be helpful."

- "2 Corinthians 12:9: 'My grace is sufficient for you, for my power is made perfect in weakness.' This text came to both of us immediately upon finding out that my husband had Parkinson's. Many times when we find ourselves thinking of the future struggles we may have to face, these words bolster us, just knowing that Christ's *power* will be made perfect in our weakness."

11

Maintaining Friendships

Two are better than one. . . . If one falls down,
his friend can help him up. But pity the man
who falls and has no one to help him up!
—Ecclesiastes 4:9-10

A letter written to Ann Landers on January 18, 1992
reads:

> *My husband, who is only 46, is terminally ill. He*
> *has been battling cancer for almost a year and*
> *unless we have a miracle, he won't live much*
> *longer. . . . [The letter addresses family and friends*
> *by adding] Where are you? Do you know how*
> *lonely we are? You were all there at the beginning*
> *when the shock was so great . . . you didn't know*
> *what to say, but you came anyway. . . . That was*
> *almost a year ago. Where have you been since? Do*
> *you know we long to hear the phone ring, to see a*
> *car in the driveway or a card in the mail? You*
> *don't have to stay long. . . . But right now we feel*
> *as if we've been abandoned. . . . The thing is, I*
> *know you'll be there at his funeral to say how*
> *sorry you are and offer to help. Then you'll disap-*
> *pear again. . . . This happens often to cancer*

> *patients and their families. . . . I don't want to*
> *leave you with the impression that we have no one*
> *around to love and care for us. There has been a*
> *nucleus of people who have been faithful from the*
> *beginning and without them, and God, we could*
> *not have come this far. But so many others who*
> *we believed really care have simply fallen by the*
> *wayside.*[1]

Anyone involved in a chronic situation knows that it can change relationships outside the family as well as within. Friends react as they do to other difficult situations. Some handle it well; others disappear. Friendships are to be treasured. Our lives are quite empty with no one with whom to share our thoughts and dreams. But it is difficult to know how to be a friend to a chronic situationer. What is the responsibility of a good friend?

Lost friendships are one of the real heartbreaks people in a chronic situation face. Friends may not call for a variety of reasons. Many, perhaps most, have an uncomfortable feeling when they are around someone who is seriously ill or injured. They might not know how to respond to a change in appearance. They may not want to face the possibility of their friend's death or their own eventual death. They may still care but don't know what to do or say. Perhaps they feel that friendship is a two-way street and they're afraid that the chronic situationer will be taking too much from them and not be able to give in return. It might simply hurt too much to see their friend in pain.

> *The greatest lie is that friendships will come*
> *automatically to us free and clear, without risking*
> *anything or doing something to pursue it. A healthy*
> *nurturing friendship demands work.—Unknown*

Keep in mind that people will stay away if they sense *you* withdrawing, which you might do without realizing it. It is easy to pull away from people out of the fear that they won't be there for you. Or you may want so much to be tough and independent that you convey to others an "I don't really need people" attitude. Lapses into these types of self-defense go with the territory of chronic illness. The important thing is not to assume automatically that your friends have made the first move in distancing themselves from you. Ask those close to you if you are giving mixed signals.

> *The best vitamin for developing friends is B1.*
> *—Unknown*

To the Chronic Situationer

Relationships really are two-way. The old saying, "To have a friend, you've got to be a friend" still applies to the person for whom a chronic medical condition has caused drastic life changes. How do you remain the kind of person who is still a true friend? You do have limitations now—in time, energy, maybe in mobility or availability. But what kind of qualities, attitudes, and habits can you still cultivate so that friendship continues to be a vital force in your life?

Choose your goals. It is true that "chronic illness does eliminate many of our choices in life, and quite understandably, we grieve for our lost opportunities. Nevertheless, some choices do remain for us, no matter how disabled we are. No matter how many dreams we have lost, we can choose to appreciate what remains and set new goals, rather than despair over our losses. We can use our remaining abilities to make a contribution, rather than dwell on our misfortunes. We must do what can be done, rather than

177

brood futilely over what can't be done. We can use our illness as a means to find a richer and more fulfilling life. The decision is ours."[2]

When asked, "How are you?" don't launch into a long detailed description of your condition. "How are you?" is a *greeting*, not a question. Some of our close friends will pursue the issue and say, "Now tell me how you *really* feel." That then gives permission to be more open. People avoid complainers and one who is wrapped up in herself. In one article, Barb Heerspink talks about her experiences with polio: "When meeting friends or acquaintances, I always greet them with a smile. I have discovered that it is important to put them at ease, and inquiring about something or someone of interest to them usually does the trick. Keeping conversation on the normal flow, instead of centered on myself or on the plight of the disabled, is of far more interest to me and to them."

Do ask for help even though it's scary. It should not be that way, but the chronic situationer usually ends up breaking the ice by calling his friends and asking if they can help in a certain way. Most people want to help and are happy if there is something concrete they can do to show their continuing friendship. They take their clues from the situationer and need guidance as to how to proceed. When Roberta Lazes' husband suffered a severe stroke, she realized that she couldn't care for him all by herself. She sent a "reaching out" letter:

> *Since Alex had his stroke, I have had caring and concern from friends and family. It has ranged from homemade soup, to reading poetry to Alex or building a ramp for him. . . . There has been*

*no end of caring, caring, caring. . . . I have not
had the energy nor the time to respond to each of
your calls, cards, or letters. We've moved into a
new stage now that Alex is home. He needs people—to play chess or checkers with—to listen to
music with—or just to sit around with. He does
physical and speech exercises (which take about
15 minutes) several times each day and needs
help with those. . . . It's hard to phrase this letter
without seeming to apply pressure. I know you're
busy with your own lives and may not be able to
come at all. Call me if you think you can fit in—in
some small way. But please understand that if I
put you off, we may be overloaded—or it may be
he has had too much company. Thanks for any
help you can give me because I surely need it. . . .
We have such a wonderful network of support
from all of you. Thanks so much from both of us."[3]*

Keep in mind that not all people are going to volunteer—
and don't feel rejected by that. People have their own needs,
pressures, and agendas of what they can or want to do.

Also keep in mind that support can dwindle over time.
When the initial crisis passes, people pick up their own
lives and their own troubles. This is normal, and you should
not feel too deeply hurt by this.

Return to work as soon as you are physically able.
Work provides satisfaction and a chance to interact with
peers. If your situation makes it impossible to return to
your former line of work, investigate the possibilities of
retraining programs within the community and possibly
prepare for another occupation. Remember that coworkers
are often unsure of what to say or do for you.

A man with MS relates that, "Using a wheelchair at work was probably the greatest challenge I have had to face. It took both my fellow employees as well as myself a lot of adjustment. . . . A person in a chair does have to make some considerable effort to put people at ease. After a while the chair became part of me and as I became more comfortable with it, so did others around me. I do think that if more able bodied adults would not be so afraid to talk to or ask questions of a wheelchair user, it would be so much easier for them."[4]

Do cultivate a sense of humor and laugh at yourself. Examine your attitude. Show others that you can see the lighter side of your situation.

Do ask others to pray for you. You can form a private prayer chain among your friends. If you're too tired or pained to pray yourself, give them a call.

Do be honest about your feelings. That helps everyone involved adapt more easily to this intrusion in your lives. Staying in touch with your emotions provides an emotional catharsis under stressful circumstances. Attend a support group and share your feelings with a small number of friends.

> *If a little help may ease*
> *The burdens of another;*
> *God give us love and care and strength*
> *To help along each other.*
> *—Anonymous*

Say "thank you" often and gracefully. None of us want to be a burden, and it certainly is a blow to our pride to need help. It isn't just the chronic situationer's problem;

the whole family may feel this way.

Anne B. Lawler in her article, "Saying Thank-you, Gracefully," relates how their friends got together and gave her and her husband, who has MS, a van with a lift. At first it was difficult for them to enjoy that wonderful gift, but then they realized that it was given out of love and not of pity.

Saying "thank you" can be followed by some act of love the chronic situationer can accomplish. This can mean getting outside yourself by praying for others, writing notes and cards, sharing stitchery items, being willing and open about disease, death, and dying, talking, listening, and encouraging others.

> *As you refresh others, you relieve your own pain. Pain is inevitable. The trick is to find ways to not let it turn into misery. So when someone sends a note, a card, or clipping, or gives me a call that boosts my spirits, it prompts me to think of ways that I can refresh and encourage others in return.*
> *—Barbara Johnson*[5]

To Those Who Offer Friendship and Support

"Helpless. This one word sums up how we often feel when someone we care about is hurting—physically or emotionally. And to be helpless is to be powerless to change, cure, or 'fix' someone or something."[6]

Volunteers come in various forms: young, old, male, female, experienced, novice, introverts, extroverts—but they all have one thing in common: They are willing to help, to do whatever it takes to help their chronic situation friend. They often act behind the scenes and away from the public eye.

> *When someone we love suffers, we suffer with that person, and we would not have it otherwise, because the suffering and the love are one, just as it is with God's love for us.*—*Frederick Buechner*

Rev. Jim R. Kok, in his article, "Ninety Percent of Helping Is Just Showing Up," tells of a middle-aged man, a leader in his church, who could not go to see his dying friend. This friend was dying without the support of his friend. Sometimes just being there—daring to show up—is the most that is required of us—even though it can be difficult.

> *A real friend never gets in your way—unless you happen to be on the way down.*—*Anonymous*

It is frightening to enter another's private world of pain. But the Christian is called and committed to respond to the suffering of a friend. "When you enter another's pain, you die for others when you move out of your comfort zone and stand close to the heartbroken, feeling helpless, weak and tongue-tied."[7]

Many friends have ministered to me and my family in diverse ways over the years. Each person did what was unique for him or her. Some played more significant roles than others, but no one person did it all. Together, all these people and their gifts and generosity formed a huge network of support. They dared to come when I had difficulty breathing. They posed as my parents and my sisters when I was in Intensive Care. They sent messages via my ICU nurses. They babysat, did laundry, brought meals, did yardwork, cleaned, provided transportation, provided money for medical expenses, shopped and aided in a host of other ways.

Without our friends and the family of God, we would not have survived. Through the love of others we have been exposed to the gracious love of our God. With the help of others, we have not allowed my disease to dominate our lives.

Practice simple awareness and sensitivity

Put yourself in the situation of your friend. Losing control of your health is scary business. How would you feel if you could no longer work, walk, or see? How would you feel if all your time and energy were being consumed in medical appointments and hospitals? How would you feel if you couldn't keep food down and you were losing your hair? How would you feel if everyone else were busy with their lives while normal activities passed you by?

Sometimes, in trying to find the positive side of a situation, we are tempted to say things like, "It's not so bad. Look at so and so. He's worse off than you. He needs a ventilator to breathe." Comparisons don't help much, and they can make you sound like you are minimizing your friend's situation. For him or her, there is no quick fix. It takes working through and it sets its own pace. Grieving over losses is a continuous process.

Greet chronic situationers the same as you do other people. If it's the first time you've met make small talk for a while and proceed to other subjects. If he wants to talk about himself, that's fine. If he doesn't, that's okay, too. Don't pity or patronize your friend.

Don't believe in myths such as "handicapped people don't have sex," or "cancer is contagious" or "deaf people are glad for peace and quiet." We may think we are intelligent adults and not prone to prejudice, but myths are taking root in us from the moment we begin to make sense out of words and meanings. If you are honest with yourself, you'll probably discover some fears and perceptions that would embarrass you if others knew about them. We have to work at not being mere products of a narrowminded society.

This is all the more reason to do some homework so that you can understand some of the basic jargon of your friend's situation. This way you can talk intelligently with her and help her make choices. Materials can be found in a library or bookstore or at a doctor's office. Ask your friend questions and she will be happy to share that information.

Learn to overcome that innate fear of illness and death that would cause you to avoid being close to a chronic situationer. When we moved to a new location, one woman saw me in church and vowed, "I'm staying away from that woman." She was scheduled to bring a meal for us and was petrified. Now she is a good friend. Chronic situationers are regular people with a few adjustments. The average person fears talking about disease, fears his or her own emotional reaction to the situation: *What if I start crying?* Most of us were apprehensive the first time we drove in a strange city or spoke in front of an audience, too. Fears are meant to be overcome.

Children are wonderful. They are spontaneous and un-inhibited in their curiosity. They take a few seconds to look over my wheelchair and assess the situation. Then they venture a question: "How come you have those wheels?"

They go on, "Do you sleep in your chair? Can you feel this? How do you go to the bathroom?" I often go to chapel and demonstrate how my wheelchair comes apart and how I use a sliding board for transfers. I shake every child's hand and they accept me as I am.

While I don't expect adults to be quite as blunt as children, I would love it if they felt as free to ask me questions.

Stay connected

It is so easy to become isolated when illness moves in to take a permanent spot in the family. The situationer is involved with "illness" type things; sometimes she is confined and really depends on others to bring the world in. Phone calls are usually welcome. When people don't want to answer the phone, they can turn it off. Having a phone prayer chain of friends and church members lends a wonderful feeling of support.

Help your friend to have a link with the outside world. Fellowship with others is healthy. Call your friend and invite him for lunch. If he cannot leave the house or hospital, bring lunch to him and fellowship while you eat. If you find an article, book, or pamphlet that speaks to his situation, give or send it. Be careful that it isn't too preachy. The fact that someone took the time and effort to cut and send an article makes your friend feel loved. Pray about the material you're giving your friend—that it will make connection with real needs. And a situationer needs to hear from time to time that others are proud of his courage and persistence in going on with his life.

Everyone needs physical affection. Babies need to be held and loved. Elderly and ill persons need touching. "Skin-hunger, some call it. The skin is the largest organ of the human body—the sensor of temperature, judger of texture, instrument of emotional contact. The skin is also the prison within which we live, the barrier which isolates us from one another—until we reach across the distance to touch another person . . . Human beings thrive on physical contact." [8] The nicest thing about a hug is that you usually can't give one without getting one.

Offer tangible help

There are endless practical ways—large and small—to be a friend to a person who is ill or disabled. Some of these suggestions take very little time but mean a lot. The beauty of helping others is that in most situations there is enough to do that you can choose what kinds of tasks suit your own schedule and gifts.

Following are just a few practical suggestions.

- If asked, go along with for medical appointments or a support group.
- Help financially if there is a need and you can afford it.
- Ask if you can help with some job or task. Simply ask, "Do you want some help?" If the person declines, respect that.
- "Call me anytime" is too general. Give your friend a couple of options and suggestions. "We'd be happy to have your kids spend Sunday with us. Have them bring play clothes and boots." Knowing that the children are cared for and entertained can relieve a worn-out parent. Including the children on trips to the zoo, museum, skating rink, or mall gets them out of the house for a while.
- Cook a dinner for the family. Give them a choice between two or three possibilities. If possible bring the meal in disposable containers or marked dishes.

Bring cookies or items that can be used in children's school lunches or to serve when visitors come.

- Help with the yardwork, household chores, or laundry.
- Offer to help with transportation, especially if children are involved in outside activities.
- Shopping errands are endless with a chronic situation in a family. Call your friend, tell him you're going shopping, and ask if there's anything he needs.
- Write encouragement in the form of a note, card, or letter. Written forms of communication can be read at the patient's convenience, and she can reread them many times. Including appropriate Scripture can often accomplish more than human words. Scripture can reveal the depths of *God's* love.
- Offer to write thank-you letters or help with correspondence. Friends and relatives need to be updated in order to pray more intelligently.
- Send flowers, balloons, reading materials, and other small gifts.
- Offer to play games or read to help pass the time.

Be an emotional support

When a person is physically ill, more than his or her physical body is affected. Without warning or permission, the emotional state gets rearranged, too. It doesn't matter how mature a person may be, or how spiritually in tune, how optimistic his outlook, or how wise or witty he is. The very fact that something is wrong with his body is going to have a physiological impact on his whole being—and mind and emotions are in the package. Whatever weaknesses a person may have had prior to the illness or accident, they remain and can become intensified. So someone prone to being fearful or pessimistic about life has a greater battle to fight. Even character strengths will get tested; eventually the most sunshiny optimist must face the reality that life has been changed permanently.

It isn't the end of the world, no matter how much it may feel that way. All kinds of people have made incredible strides in their emotional lives in the midst of what would seem to others to be impossible conditions. God has given us the ability to thrive in our minds, spirits, and emotions: "Therefore we do not lose heart. Though outwardly we are wasting away, yet inwardly we are being renewed day by day" (2 Corinthians 4:16).

Part of the equipment God has given us to weather these storms, survive and thrive, is relationships. We were never meant to go through life—its joys or trials—alone. Some strong, independent people don't learn this until they become ill or disabled. If you are the friend of a situationer, that person needs your emotional support just as much as physical/practical support. Here are some helps to keep in mind.

Be sensitive to the moods and emotions of your friend. If a person is very ill and hasn't eaten for days, it is not the time to bring food and be eating in her presence. Allow her to express her emotions—negative or positive—without feeling guilty. Don't give spiritual or medical diagnoses. If you're asked your opinion, be honest.

Respect your friend's wheelchair, hospital bed, or other medical equipment. Unless you know the person well, it is not appropriate to sit on a friend's bed. In the same way, don't lean on a person's wheelchair. If he spends a lot of time in the wheelchair, it feels like an extension of his own body; by touching the chair it feels to the person that you are in effect touching him.

Remember that fatigue is a frustrating factor to cope with. Try to be flexible and to understand if your friend must cancel plans at the last minute. Include her in plans for the next outing.

Allow your situationer friend to help *you* in some way. Everyone needs to be needed.

Offer hope. Living does not end with a serious diagnosis. Listen to your friend talk of pre-illness or pre-accident days when she had energy and strength. Be willing to talk about what the future might hold for your friend. The power of planning is terrific. Talk of your friend's child graduating from high school or marrying. Looking forward to special events gets her mind off the present pain. Stress the activities that your friend can still participate in instead of dwelling on what was lost.

Point the way to resources that may benefit your friend. These resources could be professionals in the areas of pastoral ministry, pastoral counseling, and other health-care teams that can serve as a network of caring.

There may come a time when you need to give your friend a "kick in the pants" to remind him of the blessings he still can enjoy. Gloria Chisholm defines encouragement as: "to spur one another on toward love and good deeds." At the time it may be painful, but if a kick in the pants is initiated by the Holy Spirit, it will bear fruit and be a learning experience for all involved.

And then sometimes gentleness is called for. If your friend becomes discouraged and doesn't feel that life is worthwhile, gently encourage him. At all times we have to be discerning about what our friends need most.

And we urge you, brothers, warn those who are idle, encourage the timid, help the weak, be patient with everyone.—1 Thessalonians 5:14

How to Listen

Helping your friend open up and talk about his chronic situation is one of the greatest gifts you can give. It takes directness and sensitivity to address the pain. A good listener makes direct eye contact. This tells the person that you are dedicated to listening. Listen with your whole body. Touching your friend's arm or hand also conveys sincerity.

Encourage your friend to share thoughts and feelings. Let her know you are willing to become involved in conversation and in her life.

Don't fill the silences with chatter. Look your friend in the eye, smile, hold her hand, and let her know that you care.

Use short phrases to let your friend know you are still listening. "Yes, I see your point," or "Sure, go on," are ways of encouraging conversation.

When your friend has talked for a while, restate what she has said: i.e., "I can tell that this is a heavy burden for you. How should I pray for you?" Then the person feels understood and can sift through all her feelings.

Avoid pat statements like, "Everything is going to be all right." It's better not to say anything. Sometimes everything will *not* be all right.

Don't butt in with "I know how you feel," unless you have gone through the same experience yourself. If that's the case she will appreciate your sharing how you coped.

Stay away from any statement beginning with "You should" or "You shouldn't." If you have good advice, your friend will listen and then decide whether to follow it or not. Shoulds and shouldn'ts sound and feel condescending. In the same vein, remember that this person is an adult, and she can't be comforted with a pat on the hand and "Don't worry." Try to imagine what this friend has lost.

> *It is a pity that it takes less energy to open the mouth than to close it.—Unknown*

Offer spiritual companionship.

We often neglect the spiritual aspect of life because tied in with spirituality is the idea of mortality. Some people assume that if we want to pray with a sick person, it must be close to the "end"—and the person is dying. It's unfortunate that some people don't receive prayer until that point. Prayer is meant to be our strength *while we're alive, while we have things to do and be.* It's important that you find ways of being a spiritual support to your situationer friend. How rewarding and encouraging it is to have people come in and pray just as naturally and lovingly as they carry on conversations or other tasks in life.

Prayer is a major tool for supporting a person who is ill or disabled. It may go without saying, but this is a time when it is essential to maintain contact with God. When I'm too pained or weak to pray, my family and friends do it for me. Pray for specifics and expect that God will answer in specifics. During one hospitalization my friends prayed that the nurses would be able to find an IV vein without trying four or five times. A nurse found a vein on the first try and that IV lasted five days—a small miracle.

Several times my support group of seven women has visited me in the hospital. We all join hands and pray together. Being bathed in prayer gave me the courage to go on.

However, if you're going to pray and use Scripture, do it appropriately. One day, when I was very pained and weak, a friend waltzed into my hospital room and brightly said, "You know, Marcia, what Romans 8:28 says, 'And we know that in all things God works for the good of those who love him, who have been called according to his purpose.' " I believe that verse in my heart but I know the verse does not say that all things are good. As Barbara Johnson says, "All the promises of God are there and they're real and true, but right now you're bleeding, you're raw and hurting. You have to hang on to those promises even if they don't seem to work for you at the moment." [9]

I knew my friend meant well, but it would have been more helpful to me at that point if she had just held my hand and prayed with me.

People who are ill often have just enough energy to do what they *must* do, like eat and cooperate with the nurses, technicians, and doctors who treat them. Although we may appreciate reading material, sometimes we're just too exhausted to hold it up and read for ourselves. Ask your friend from time to time if he wants to be read to. And don't restrict your reading to "spiritual" material like the Bible or inspirational books. Poetry, humor, essays, fiction—all minister to our emotions and spirits in their own way and time.

Support your friend if she wants to be anointed with oil and prayed over by the minister and church elders. A friend of mine, who has MS, was anointed as it speaks of in the book of James. Her MS didn't disappear, but she received the gift of endurance and was bathed in the treatment of prayer.

Never indicate to an ill person that the reason he wasn't healed is because he doesn't have enough faith. It is humanly impossible for you to know how much faith another person has. Even if you have a theory about it, keep it to yourself. God gives us the faith we need when we need it, as we turn to him.

Hospital and Home Visits

Visiting someone in a hospital or at home can be somewhat frightening—not just for patients but for their visitors, too. Developing skills in this area can help those who are hurting.

Be prepared. Find out from a family member or a close friend if visitors are wanted. Some people need time for undisturbed recovery. Then call first. During the day, patients are often taken from their rooms for treatments. Patients at home may have a home health care nurse or a physical therapist working with them. Make sure you arrive at a convenient time. Stay away if you have a cold or infection that can be transmitted to the patient. Pray before you go that you will be a blessing and show your friend love and concern.

Keep it short. Don't make the visit such a social event that the patient must act as host/hostess. Visiting is hard work for a patient and can leave him tired. If he appears to be fatigued, leave. Make frequent visits, but keep them brief. If you can't visit often, call to stay in touch. Call frequently if a friend is hospitalized a long distance from home.

Let the patient set the agenda. Be an active listener. If the patient wants to talk about medical fears, lend a sympathetic ear. Listen to what she has to say without being judgmental. When there is quiet, the patient often begins to talk about what is really going on inside. If your friend is very sad and down, be willing to cry with her.

Don't show shock at the way your friend looks. A negative response from a visitor can be upsetting. Be upbeat, supportive, and honest in your conversation. Don't add to the patient's worries. Humor can help battle a chronic situation if it is done tactfully. A funny card, a silly toy, a book of jokes can be uplifting.

Unless medical procedures prohibit, treat the patient as you always have. If you've always greeted with a kiss or a friendly hug, don't change. Touch conveys love and concern. Ask questions about the results of tests or surgery and how the patient feels about it. Be willing to hear about the pain and fatigue. But don't force sharing either.

If you bring a gift, be sure it's appropriate. Plants and flowers are not allowed in Intensive Care areas. Food generally is not a good idea for a patient on a special diet. Also, some patients have allergies—avoid bringing or wearing strong cologne and perfumes.

Be prepared to lead in prayer if your friend wishes. Holding hands and praying together can be a piece of heaven on earth. Pray for courage and hope for the patient and his family. Use Scripture appropriately. Ask if the patient would like you to read a short passage from the Bible. Read passages that are full of hope and encouragement.

Offer practical help. Ask your friend if there's anything he might need help with like errands or shopping. Make yourself available.

> *Both truth and communication begin with a simple gesture: touch, the authentic voice of feeling. The loving touch, like music, often utters the things that cannot be spoken—nothing need be said, for everything is understood.—Ashley Montagu*

A chronic situationer highly values the visits of his friends. These expressions and reminders of love give much encouragement when emotional resources are running low.

The Role of the Church

The purpose of the church is to be united in love. Colossians 3:12 reads: "Therefore, as God's chosen people, holy and dearly loved, clothe yourselves with compassion, kindness, humility, gentleness and patience."

The sick or disabled are and always will be a central concern of the body of Christ. The church visits, comforts, prays for and ministers to the those in need. But often, as Rev. Jim Kok says, "church groups see their roles as spiritual caregivers, helping people with their soul problems but not with their illness." [10]

> *Sharing our suffering with other Christians is*
> *one of the best responses to suffering.—Unknown*

Rev. Kok goes on to say that the church should not care just for the soul of a member, but also for the physical and mental aspects of that person's life. The church should see each person as a soul-body unity. Healing comes from medicine and surgery, but also from love and encouragement of fellow Christians.

It's not uncommon for church members to become impatient in the case of a chronic situationer. Perhaps a group of people will come in and pray for healing. What they want and expect is healing *right now* when, in fact, this seldom happens. Christians in this instant-gratification culture have much to learn about God's process of healing. We must learn what it is to pray persistently and with hope and how we can have faith and at the same time take a posture of waiting for God's answers. What often happens is that a group of pray-ers receive an answer of "No," or "Not now," and they became frustrated and angry. Sometimes—more often than we want to admit—church members actually blame the person who's sick: He wasn't really trying hard enough to improve his situation. Or, her faith is weak, or there's some unconfessed sin. All of these accusations take place because as a church we are quite unpracticed at waiting on and trusting God. This kind of anger and blame can drive a person out of the church and away from the love and concern of God's people.

It's important for church people—and particularly church leaders—to remember that the chronically ill or disabled person is just as important to church life as the member who volunteers many service hours per week. All are part of God's kingdom on earth. Joni Eareckson Tada says, "God doesn't want us for the sake of things we can do for Him. He wants our love. He wants our fellowship. He wants our worship. And any of us—rich or poor, healthy or ill—can offer Him this." [11]

> *My family has experienced the love and support of a caring congregation. For that we thank God. We pray that many others who need that assistance may also receive this gift of God, who alone truly understands.—Dr. John Kromminga*

Everyone has a spiritual gift, and the church needs to provide opportunities for the situationer to contribute to church life. A disease or disability does not excuse anyone from his or her obligations and responsibilities. Getting involved offers the opportunity to become acquainted with fellow church members. Soon the situationer is no longer just "that woman in a wheelchair." A chronic situationer can be an excellent listener and confidante to those going through similar experiences.

Don't forget to consider physical aspects of church life. Is your church accessible for the physically disabled? Are there signers for the deaf? To feel a oneness of the Spirit, the situationer needs to worship, sing, and fellowship with other believers. But physical barriers can keep all that from happening if we're not alert to them.

Churches should establish programs that train laypersons to minister to the needs of the congregation. One of these programs is the "Stephen Ministry." These volunteers spend fifty hours learning, "the art of listening, sensing other's feelings, compassionate assertiveness, maintaining confidentiality, crisis theory and intervention, effective telephone care, praying with people and finding help in the Bible." These volunteers are taught "to recognize needs requiring professional help and how to refer the individual to appropriate counselors, physicians or community agencies." [12]

For more information, contact:

Rev. Glenn Bolsclair
Stephen Ministries
8016 Dale
St. Louis, MO 63117-1449
(314) 645-5511

Stephen Ministries are especially appropriate for those people who have the spiritual gift of mercy.

Those in the church with the gift of administration can organize prayer chains, meals, laundry, transportation to church events, medical appointments, shopping, household work, etc.

Others have the gift of giving. Help with medical expenses, traveling expenses, and insurance premiums is always appreciated.

The Fragile Balance

As Christians we are called upon to love others. And as Christians, we are called upon to be vulnerable to others. This means that friends and family and church members have the responsibility to pay attention to the needs of those people in their spheres of influence who suffer from chronic disease or disability. And it also means that the chronic situationer must dare to make her needs known, must not be ashamed of weakness and pain but give others the opportunity to help and be involved. People who are well must move beyond their fears and apprehensions about illness and death, and people who are ill must move beyond their immediate medical needs and find ways to keep living and contributing.

All of this represents a fragile balance. Such a balance is easily upset. It calls for everyone involved to practice awareness and honesty. It takes work from all sides to keep our relationships with others strong and healthy. But the good part of all this is that we learn the deeper lessons of love. Friendships purified in the fires of illness become lasting and wonderful gifts.

Part Four

Realities of a
Terminal Condition

12

Important Decisions

*"For my thoughts are not your thoughts,
neither are your ways my ways," declares the
LORD.—Isaiah 55:8*

Recently a study of world health revealed that half the human race is physically ill. This means that one and three quarter billion people are suffering bodily disease. This figure includes Third World countries who have very little medical technology. People in many of these countries face famine, drought, floods, volcanoes, earthquakes, and other disasters. If these people had better food, sanitation, and medical care, the figure would decline.

In the United States, we have more access to new medications and surgical procedures. But, in spite of all these new advances, the science of medicine never catches up in the race against illness. As bacteria are overcome, viruses arise. While tuberculosis and pneumonia still exist, heart disease and cancer become the new killers. Typhoid and polio cases decline but AIDS becomes the newest disease to overcome.

Each time a new defense is discovered against an old enemy of humanity, a new enemy springs up. We spend billions of dollars on health care, but the number of physically ill does not decrease.

"For all our streamlined machinery, our miracle drugs, our surgical skills, the doctor can find no medical cure for perhaps half, or more than half, of the sufferers who come to him for health."[1]

"It is estimated that in the next 50 years, the number of elderly in this country will double and that Americans over 65 will constitute more than 20 percent of the population. This group of the 'very old' is expected to triple in the next 50 years, from 2 million to 6 million people."[2]

New kind of dying

What does all of this mean? It means that as people get older, they may face progressive decline in health and often a *prolonged dying process*. A 1987 report in *The New England Journal of Medicine* estimated that nearly 80 percent of the medical expenses throughout a person's life will be spent in the last two or three months of that life.

Before the 1950s, many people died naturally at home without technical means and surrounded by family and loved ones. When the person's heart stopped and he could no longer breathe, he was pronounced dead. Today, most deaths occur in hospitals or nursing homes. Dying is no longer a simple process.

Decisions about life-and-death issues have become more complex in the last thirty years. We are involved in more medical options—yet there is little to tell us specifically how we should make these bio-ethical decisions.

The big questions

This country's development of sophisticated technology, which can save and prolong human life, has also left us with many questions, such as: What is life? When is a person dead? Should a person go on a life-support system? Should a person cling to life at all costs? What is "passive" euthanasia? What is "active" euthanasia? Should one donate his organs for transplants? What is a living will?

We all know people who have been and are faced with these questions. The "right" answers are not always crystal clear.

> *Be to the world a sign that while we as Christians do not have all the answers, we do care about the questions.—Billy Graham*

What Is Life?

First of all, human life must be considered in terms of its relationship with God, the Creator. Genesis 2:7 reads, "The LORD God formed the man from the dust of the ground and breathed into his nostrils the breath of life, and the man became a living being." We are made in the image of God, and that makes life precious. He knows all about our birth, life, and death. Life starts with conception. A human is distinct as a separate entity. Body, soul, and spirit are combined and intertwine to function as a unit.

Can there be any meaning to life if one is kept alive on life-support but cannot respond in any way?

What happens when a body organ fails? Often a machine or a transplant can take over for the failed organ. Isn't this person still a human being? Aren't we morally obligated to protect and care for him or her?

We know that certain tissues can be preserved for months after removal from human patients. When reimplanted, they live and function again. A leg muscle can be revived eight or ten hours after death. Nails, hair, and parts of the skin continue to grow for days after death. Is this considered life? No.

When a person's brain ceases to function, the body itself—even if kept alive by machines—is not a person anymore.

There is no personality. When death occurs, the body returns to dust and the spirit goes to its eternal destiny.

What Is Death?

"The brain, which is the most sensitive of the organs to toxic influences, including lack of oxygen, is vital for the somatic motor and sensory functions, the higher mental activities and the emotions."[3]

Death occurs when: 1) breathing and heartbeat stop; 2) the irreversible cessation of all brain activity occurs, even if the body could be kept functioning on high-tech machines.

Dr. Kenneth E. Schemmer, in his book *Between Life and Death,* states that "we can actually pinpoint when a human being is really dead. We no longer need to worry about pulling the plug too soon because we can now test to see if the neocortex is still functioning."[4] The neocortex is the part of the brain that distinguishes human beings from animals. In some cases, the brain stem can be functioning because it controls the heart and lungs. The President's Commission on Foregoing Life Sustaining Treatment recommends using the term "permanent loss of consciousness." In this condition, the brain tissue is dead. That person is permanently gone.

Organ Transplants

> *The moral test of government is how it treats those who are in the dawn of life—the children: those who are in the twilight of life—the aged: those who are in the shadows of life—the sick, the needy and the handicapped.—Hubert Humphrey*

An April 1, 1992 article by Dan Anderson in the *Inland Valley Daily Bulletin* calls our attention to a baby born without a brain neocortex. Anencephalic infants, like Theresa Ann Campo Pearson, often die within hours or days of birth. Ethicists have been debating whether organs removed from an anencephalic infant can be used as transplants. Should the baby be on life support so that the organs may be used for transplants?

Each year about 3,000 babies are born with anencephalia. None of them have any feelings, even to pain. It is estimated that the need for donor hearts and kidneys is between 400 and 500, and 1,000 livers are needed. These anencephaly babies could provide these organs. But according to the law in most states, both breathing and heartbeat need to cease in order for someone to be declared dead.

Dan Anderson's article goes on to say that hospitals nationwide have avoided the issue by simply not establishing any policies or programs regarding organ harvesting from anencephalic babies. Most infant organ transplants come from children experiencing Sudden Infant Death Syndrome or accidents.

Adult organ transplanting also presents difficult questions. We have established that the neocortex function is necessary for a human body to be a person. When death is sudden and unexpected, or the person was previously active and in good health, all resuscitative measures should be attempted. Resuscitative measures are not indicated for persons who have died as a result of chronic debilitative disease, widespread malignancies, those in comas, and those with crushing wounds to the head or body.

It becomes complicated when the person has given his permission for removal of one or more of his organs for transplantation. Then the question is: should this person be kept alive by machine until the organs have been removed? By law, no organ should be removed unless all the criteria of death has been confirmed. When the time comes that all hope of existence for the donor has been abandoned by the doctor, he informs the members of the family and the respirator is turned off. Then the transplant team proceeds with their work.

Dr. Schemmer says, "The cost of organ transplantation continues to rise so the value of the whole transplantation program comes into question. Should we be spending so much money on so few people when so many die of common disease?" [5]

Questions abound. Will it be only the rich who can afford transplants? What if one person's body has already rejected one or two organs—should someone else have a chance? Who is eligible for a transplant—the person who has the most chance of recovery?

Donating useable organs is a way to contribute something unselfishly to others even in our death. More information can be obtained by writing or calling:

> The Living Bank
> P.O. Box 6725
> Houston, TX 77265
> 1-800-528-2971

What about Life Support?

This country's sophisticated technology that can save lives can also prolong life. With the current trend, critically ill and injured people will be put on some kind of a life-support system. Society has demanded high technology treatments in large medical centers. The question is always asked:

"Did they do everything possible?" Many doctors view death as defeat, and they talk about "losing a patient."

Dr. Schemmer writes, "The development of the life-support dilemma occurred out of a desire to help return sick and infirmed people to normal health. There was no real thought of prolonging the dying stage—patients fear that they will get stuck on a life-support system without meaningful personal contact. That's what denies them their sense of personal worth and dignity, not necessarily the machine itself."[6]

The patient is not being morbid if he discusses a treatment plan and what the quality of life will be if he has certain treatments and procedures. Knowing that he will be treated according to his desires can provide tremendous peace of mind. He has the right to refuse life-prolonging treatment if he is able to understand the consequences of choices and make rational decisions.

Some of the questions that should be asked before life-prolonging treatment is used:

1. What will the treatment accomplish? Will it help the patient get well or ease the pain of the illness?
2. What are the odds that it will work? What are the side-effects of this treatment?
3. Does it matter if the patient refuses treatment now and later changes his mind?
4. Is this what the patient wants? For many people, life on a support system is intolerable. Can the patient die with dignity while on a support system?

Situations are not always black and white.

In the early 1980s, two Kaiser Permanente Harbor City doctors were accused of murder for withdrawing life support from a comatose patient. The case was thrown out of court.

In the last few years we've read much about the questions involved in life support. One man asked the courts to allow him to turn off his respirator and they agreed, but he has changed his mind.

Then we have a man who suffered from emphysema, heart disease, and lung cancer—hospital personnel restrained his arms to prevent him from pulling the plug.

A young Long Beach couple kept their brain-dead baby on life support for eight months before agreeing to its removal. The parents believed that a miracle could revive their child.

Often families get involved in life-support decisions because they have hope that their loved one will improve. One family said yes to a respirator, feeding tube, tracheotomy, to anti-seizure medication and antibiotics—all within the first ten days.

Janet Kaye, author of "The Long Goodbye," says, about her father's illness, "Anyone who has spent time with a loved one in an intensive-care unit knows that an uncertain prognosis can be interpreted as a cause for hope. At the time our decisions were made, there was, we believed, a great deal of hope for our father."[7] Janet goes on to say that her mother now owes $200,000 because her father is being kept alive on a respirator and a feeding tube. "For us, the issues go on and on and on. Like Dad, we are living on hold."[8]

The AMA estimates that medical institutions artificially sustain 10,000 permanently unconscious individuals.

When you must make a life-support decision, try to be content with your decisions and patient with others. It is a very sad experience to go through, and you may feel all alone. Remember that you are not the only ones struggling to make these decisions. Getting the opinion of other relatives about discontinuing life-support for your loved one can be very helpful. Hospital chaplains and other spiritual counselors are experienced in these circumstances. Praying for direction is especially important.

Getting as much medical information as possible removes some of the fear from these decisions. Ask the nursing staff and the doctors what the tubes and machines are doing and what would happen if they were removed.

Follow the expressed wishes of the patient, whether verbal or in writing (Living Will and Durable Power of Attorney). If the patient is terminally ill and expressed his desire for nature to take its course, that wish should be honored. Think of what you would want done if you were the patient in these circumstances.

Once decisions are made, be at peace with them and take comfort from knowing that you have loved and cared for your loved one in life and in death.

What Is a Living Will?

The Living Will movement arose primarily from an able-bodied person's concern that he would be kept alive longer than he wanted to be. A Living Will may contain an advance directive of your wish not to be connected to life-support equipment. If it is judged that you are hopelessly and terminally ill, your wishes will be carried out.

In November, 1991, the Patient Self Determination Act required all hospitals and extended care facilities to ask patients on admission if they have an advanced directive. A copy of one of these documents can be found in Appendix A.

Discussing an advance directive with one's family, close friends, or religious advisor is an important step in the process of writing a Living Will.

A Living Will tells your relatives what you want done—or do not want done—should you get so sick you cannot tell the doctors yourself. For example, you can say under what conditions you want life-support systems to stay or go; or whether or not you want chemotherapy, surgery, or radiation treatments for cancer. It tells whether or not you want doctors to get your heart started if it stops or to have a brain hemorrhage treated.

A 1988 study reported that 80 percent of Americans would want life-support systems disconnected should they lapse into an irreversible coma. However, only 9 percent had prepared a written directive making their wishes clear. Since then, because of all the publicity, a much higher number of persons have written Living Wills.

Items That Should Be Addressed Regarding a Living Will

1. In all states, the Living Will must be prepared in advance of the situation and at a time when the patient is competent and of sound mind. You must be at least eighteen years of age to make a Living Will.
2. In some states, the Living Will is not in effect during pregnancy.
3. The majority of states require that only certain people may witness a Living Will. The witnesses should not

---

be related to you by blood or marriage, entitled to part of your estate if you die, be your attending doctor or an employee of that doctor or the health care facility where you are a patient.

4. All the laws permit the signer to change his mind. You can do this by destroying the Living Will, writing down your intent, or telling someone. Make sure you tell your doctor.

5. Most of the laws specify that the Living Will can only be implemented *after* your physician and one other doctor have certified that the "living will" is not an instrument for casual suicide.

6. If your doctor doesn't want to honor a Living Will, he is required by most laws to find another doctor or health-care facility where your wishes will be carried out.

7. Keep your Living Will in a safe place in your home. Give a photocopy to a family member, close friend, doctor, and the hospital. It is your responsibility to make sure your doctor and hospital have your Living Will in their files.

8. A Living Will should not affect your insurance policies.

9. Samples of Living Wills are available and can be obtained from a lawyer, the local medical society, or the social services department of a community hospital. Living Will forms can be obtained at no cost by writing to:
   The Society for the Right to Die
   250 West 57th St.
   New York, NY 10107

10. Doctors and courts are not bound by the law to honor a Living Will, but most doctors respect a Living Will as a lawful request. It is a valuable factor in the doctor's thinking about how to handle your dying. The Living Will will give the doctor protection from lawsuits by relatives after your death.

11. When hospitalized or in a nursing home, make sure that the Living Will is fully understood by the staff. DNR (do not resuscitate) or No Code Blue should be written on your chart to avoid life-saving devices.

Dr. Doron Weber, direction of communications at the Concern for Dying and Society for the Right to Die office there, says that there has been an influx in the number of requests for Living Wills. She said, "We have sent out 800,000 Living Wills since the Supreme Court decisions in the Nancy Cruzan case last June (she died December 26, 1990). This office pioneered the Living Will in 1967 and there are now 41 states which have standard Living Wills." [9]

Disabled Americans are making Living Wills very specific. They are interested in having a Living Will to *protect* their lives from premature discontinuation of medical help, as much as protecting themselves from unwanted intrusive medical procedures.

My Living Will very specifically states that when I no longer can breathe on my own, I *want* to be put on a respirator so I can live, not die. I have been on a respirator before and came back, and I don't want anyone giving up on me before I'm ready. Many disabled persons do not consider respirators or feeding tubes to be monstrous machines. They consider them as normal ways to sustain life.

Some Living Wills say they want everything turned off except the IV. Others want to be kept pain free. Still others say they want no artificial support systems—period.

Durable Power of Attorney

A more potent document than the Living Will is the Durable Power of Attorney for Health Care, which in different forms is available in all American states. Here you assign someone else the power to make health-care decisions if and when you cannot.

As of today, however, it works only for passive euthanasia (the withdrawing of treatment) and does not empower anybody to perform euthanasia (helping to die).

Carold Gill, a disability psychologist says, "Durable Power of Attorney is a superior measure [to the Living Will] because that person can act for you when you become incompetent and can make any of a wide range of decisions about you. The Living Will only spells out contingencies in specific situations; if your health is such that you fall into another category, the Living Will can't dictate what would happen." [10]

A copy of a Durable Power of Attorney form can be obtained by writing:

Concern for Dying
250 West 57th St.
New York, NY 10107

> *In a society that can't agree when human life begins, it's no surprise that we have trouble deciding when it should end. If you think the abortion issue was emotional, just wait until we get fully into euthanasia and death.—Margaret Battin, Philosophy professor, University of Utah*

What Is Euthanasia?

There are many issues facing doctors today. Dr. Kenneth E. Schemmer notes that doctors are trained to heal, not kill. He says that in "affirming his Hippocratic Oath, I promised that 'I will give no deadly medicine to anyone if asked, nor suggest any such counsel; furthermore, I will not give to a woman an instrument to produce abortion.'" [11]

The whole issue of euthanasia is centuries old. The Germans, between 1921 and 1944, practiced genocide under the supervision of medical doctors, claiming it was an act of compassion. Anyone who was deemed "life unworthy of life" was killed in the name of healing.

The word *euthanasia* means "a good and peaceful death." Everyone agrees about that definition, but that is where the agreement stops. Killing in the name of healing is how the whole abortion issue began. Women who had become pregnant were interviewed. If two psychiatrists agreed that the woman would have deep psychological problems if she had the baby, then a gynecologist performed a therapeutic abortion. The victims of rape and incest were the next group to have abortions. Why should a pregnant teenager be forced to carry the product of a brief sexual encounter? These attitudes have led to abortion as we know it today.

If fetuses are not persons, then should we treat severely handicapped babies? Are retarded people created in God's image and useful in society? Are the disabled worthy of life? What about the elderly?

In Holland (the only country that allows active euthanasia) family physicians commit over 5,000 euthansia killings a year. The law protects physicians from prosecution and a doctor is not obligated to consult parents or guardians of a minor when the sick child asks to die and doesn't want the parents involved.

Everyone was watching last November when "Initiative 119" was included on the Washington state ballot. This initiative called for physicians to legally help terminally ill patients who want to end their lives by prescribing lethal drugs.

News reports showed that the pro-euthanasia group raised $900,000 in Washington trying to get "Initiative 119" passed. The anti-euthanasia groups such as The National Right to Life Committee only raised $150,000 to battle the proposed law.

Anti-euthanasia doctors say that this legislation, although it was defeated, has tremendous implications. It could open the door for nonvoluntary euthanasia for those deemed "life unworthy of life." It would legalize suicides assisted by physicians. The eerie part is that 46 percent of the voters approved of this initiative.

Legislatures in most states have enacted or are considering enacting statutes that are entitled "death with dignity," "natural death," and "right to die."

In June 1990, a retired pathologist from Michigan gave the use of his "suicide machine" to a woman who had sought his help to avoid the horrors of Alzheimer's disease. She pushed a button and died.

In October 1991, "Dr. Death" (as Dr. Kevorkian has been called) helped two women die on cots in a rustic cabin in the Bald Mountain area of Michigan. One woman had a mask over her face for breathing carbon monoxide from a gas bottle on the floor. The other woman was connected by hypodermic needle to a chemical solution.

In Michigan, the law on doctor-assisted suicide is unclear. Dr. Kevorkian's medical license has been suspended, but "Dr. Death" says he will continue to assist suicides even if he loses his license. Some of the controversy stems from the fact that these women were not terminally ill by some definitions.

In April 1991, a book aptly titled *Final Exit* became #1 on the New York Times' best-seller list. *Final Exit,* by Derek Humphry and published by the Hemlock Society, gives explicit advice on how one can commit suicide painlessly. Cheryl K. Smith, staff attorney for the Hemlock Society, says that "*Final Exit* is designed for and marketed toward the terminally ill." [12]

Controversy has swirled around the publication of the suicide manual because experts fear that it will be misused by people who are depressed or who might even commit murder. Others believe that it is a loud protest against the medical profession for allowing terminally ill patients to suffer.

The fact that *Final Exit* shot to the top of the best-seller list is an indication of how critical the issue of euthanasia has become in our society. Derek Humphry wrote an earlier book about how he helped his first wife, Jean, take her life when she was terminally ill. This British author said in a telephone interview that people are "tired of ethical debate among the theologians and philosophers. There's tremendous control and choice over one's dying."

Attempted suicide is not a crime punishable by law but assisted suicide is against the law (a felony) and is punishable. About 30,000 people in the United States commit suicide each year, and that statistic is by no means the world's highest.

Passive euthanasia

Passive euthanasia is commonly known as "pulling the plug." It involves the disconnection of life-support equipment. It allows nature to take its course. There is unlikely to be much legal or ethical trouble here so long as you have signed a Living Will and Durable Power of Attorney for Health Care. Both these documents express your medical wishes.

> *Death is inconvenient. In today's era of microwave meals and instant communications, any condition which tends to drag on is viewed as inconvenient. We don't want to endure the suffering process with our loved ones. We want instant death like we want instant breakfast.*
> —*Audrey T. Hingly*[13]

Active euthanasia

When a person takes steps to end his life, whether he handles the action himself or gets assistance from another person, it is termed *active euthanasia*.

Most physicians and medical organizations maintain that doctors should not participate in active euthanasia. The AMA's bioethical opinions condone withdrawing life supports in hopeless cases. They also say that the doctor should not intentionally cause death.

Should relatives of a person in an irreversible coma be allowed to tell doctors to remove all life-sustaining devices, including feeding tubes? Should a doctor be allowed to help a person end her life if she has a fatal illness? Does someone who is terminally ill have the right to end her life?

What does religion say about euthanasia?

Religious leaders are divided on the issue of euthanasia. Experts believe that euthanasia will be the major bioethical and social issue of the 1990s.

An October 1991 *Los Angeles Times* article by Russell Chandler reports, "As life expectancy continues to advance life beyond the ability of medical science to provide a comfortable existence, the medical community, lawmakers, ethicists and religious leaders will have to fashion guidelines about euthanasia that they can live with." [14]

The 1.6 million-member United Church of Christ decided that euthanasia and suicide should be options for terminally ill people. The Synod declared that a seriously ill person has the right to take his own life, and his family has a right to withhold artificial life-support systems and terminate his life.

Several other denominations, including the Presbyterian Church (U.S.A.), are leaning toward the individual's right to control his or her death. In the Episcopal Church, active euthanasia is under wide discussion.

The Islamic faith prohibits euthanasia of any kind. Muslims believe that a person does not own himself. He is entrusted to God, and the taking of life is the right of the one who gives it.

The Roman Catholic tradition emphasizes no moral obligation "to use all available medical procedures in every set of circumstances." But the bishops condemn euthanasia as a "lethal, violent and unacceptable way of terminating care for the infirm." [15]

The United Methodist Church maintains that "every person as a creation of God . . . has the right to die with dignity, free of pain, suffering and humiliation." [16]

The Jewish tradition believes that you allow life to take its course: "you neither foreshorten nor prolong it." But individual rabbis may disagree. Rabbi Harvey Field says, "I believe that where there is clearly a terminal situation and the quality of life has deteriorated and will continue to deteriorate, the person really ought to have the choice in determining how he or she wishes to die." [17]

Lewis Smedes, professor at Fuller Graduate School of Psychology in Pasadena, says that few parties on either side of the euthanasia issue appeal directly to Bible passages for support. There weren't respirators in Bible times. Dr. Smedes feels that we should appeal more to the general scriptural principles of compassion, human dignity, and worth. He also emphasizes the need "to hear special signals from God." The words of Ecclesiastes 12:7 indicate when it may be time to let "the dust [return] to the ground it came from, and the spirit [return] to God who gave it."

The American Hospital Association estimates that last year 70 percent of the 6,000 daily deaths in the United States were "somehow timed or negotiated with all concerned parties privately concurring on withdrawal of some death-delaying technology or not even starting it in the first place." [18]

More often in the last few years, clergy are being called to offer advice and counsel regarding life-support and euthanasia.

Hospice staff members say that those in terminal stages of life no longer ask to be able to end their lives after they know that someone will love and care for them and that they will have adequate pain control.

For the Christian, life is never meaningless. In all the gray areas of euthanasia, we need to see and feel God's guidance. We can rest in that comfort. He knows what is best for us.

Encouragement along the Way

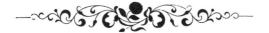

*O*ffer your bodies as living sacrifices, holy and pleasing to God—this is your spiritual act of worship. Do not conform any longer to the pattern of this world, but be transformed by the renewing of your mind. Then you will be able to test and approve what God's will is—his good, pleasing and perfect will.
—Romans 12:1-2

13

Death and Dying

Even though I walk through the valley of the shadow of death, I will fear no evil, for you are with me; your rod and your staff, they comfort me.—Psalm 23:4

A victim of chronic illness or permanent disability faces his or her mortality sooner than most people do. You have been forced to acknowledge that your body is a frail entity, and that your control over its processes is very limited. A number of chronic situations are mild enough in nature that the person can live a fairly normal life for many years; it is amazing how full and long a life can be maintained by proper care and a healthy lifestyle.

But, on the other hand, for many situationers death looms close and can shadow everything else. For this reason, this chapter and the epilogue are necessary. If you suffer from a disease that will likely not endanger your life for years to come, you may not feel compelled to read further. That's fine. In one sense, though, death and dying should be faced and thought about by every person, well or ill. A car accident or undetected infection could change everything in a matter of hours.

Our society is not comfortable with death. We seldom talk about it with those who are near death. And so we are ill-prepared to deal with it when it comes. This chapter is designed to help you look at this aspect of chronic illness with candor, objectivity, and some sense of power.

A technical definition of *dying* is: "a natural process involving the progressive degeneration of those body functions essential to maintain life." Death is not just the end of breathing or the moment a person's heart stops, but a process. In a sense all human bodies are in this process. It is another event in life and as natural as birth. When people die of old age, the body's organs are worn out and eventually cease to function. Drug treatment and other medical techniques and treatments can merely postpone the dying process.

> *It is only when we truly understand that we have a limited time on earth that we'll live each day to the fullest.—Elisabeth Kübler-Ross*

To Tell or Not to Tell

When there is a diagnosis of a terminal disease, should the patient be told the truth? It is always difficult to confront a patient after a terminal diagnosis has been made. In the past many physicians would tell the family but keep the truth from the patient—if the doctor thought the patient was unable to handle the news. More and more physicians are becoming sensitive to their patients' needs and can quite successfully make the patient aware of a serious diagnosis without taking all hope away from him. A constant procession of new drugs, treatments, and techniques often make it possible for the doctor, patient, and family to do significant battle against the disease.

Of course, one of the first questions asked by the patient is, "How long do I have to live?" As important as this question is to us, we must not be disillusioned about the doctor's ability to answer it. A whole collection of variables makes the doctor's prediction an educated guess at best. If you allow your physician to be honest about what he does and doesn't know, that will ease tension for everybody. Not knowing when we will die is simply one more reminder that, ultimately, our life and death are God's call.

> *The final test of our lives will not be how much we have lived but how we have lived, not how tempestuous our lives have been, but how much bigger, better and stronger these trials have left us. Not how much money, fame or fortune we have laid up here on earth but how many treasures we have laid up in heaven.*—Megeddo Message

Medical Attitudes toward the Dying

To give maximal care to the dying in the hospital or nursing care center, the medical staff should examine their own feelings about death. They are just as vulnerable as the rest of us, and they need to work through their own issues regarding death and dying before they can care well for terminal patients.

"Death education is too late in the hospital room where the verdict 'terminal illness' is announced. Death education has become part of the curriculum of medical and nursing schools so the physician and nurse can give leadership in helping the dying patient face the normal and ultimate in human experience." [1] These courses are helping medical students reach a better understanding of the dying process.

Medical personnel will sometimes even deny the existence of terminally ill patients on their ward. One head nurse was proud of her record of twenty years with no deaths while she was in charge; they died on the next shift.

227

One sensitive physician has spoken of how difficult it is for physicians to deal with their dying patients. It is emotionally painful for them. Some physicians find the strength to work, grieve, and to be sympathetic. Other doctors isolate themselves and may respond with disgust, anger, disappointment, and a feeling that they have failed.

Many times, nurses become the most important link with life for dying patients. Nurses should talk to the dying and by touching them express warmth and caring. Nurses assigned to areas in which death is a common occurrence need to share their feelings and reactions with others, to obtain needed support.

One nurse put her feelings into words: "I still have difficulty at times coming up with the 'right words' to say to a patient or a family member at the time when the patient is dying or has died. I have found that being a good listener or just being there with the person can be a meaningful gesture."

With so many demands on her physical and emotional energies, a nurse can distance herself from the patient. She may come in the room of a dying patient to check the IV, suction apparatus, or to monitor other equipment. None of these activities force a nurse to touch the patient. It can become a quite cold and clinical relationship, if the nurse so chooses. Of course it is impossible to spend hours holding the hand of each and every patient. Patients have no reason to expect unlimited time from their nurses. But they should be able to expect physical contact from time to time, a few moments of lingering to talk with the patient and worried family members. Caring is not so much a matter of time clocked in as it is a posture of real concern. Especially when we are dying, the warmth of someone's touch and a pair of caring eyes that are not afraid to meet ours—this should not be too much to expect from our caregivers.

A Word about "Untouchables"

A patient should be treated with dignity and respect regardless of the reason for his or her terminal condition. Caregivers and medical personnel should heed this axiom especially in a time when so many people are dying stigmatized deaths. Many terminal patients now suffer from AIDS, and the fact that this disease is often—though certainly not always—transmitted sexually should make no difference in the quality of the victim's medical care.

When a person is facing his or her own death, you can be sure that there is plenty of self-evaluation going on. Most of us are well aware of our failings; if any kind of moral help is called for, it is most likely forgiveness and support. This is not a time for other persons to be passing judgment; it is certainly not appropriate for medical personnel to do so.

How a Physician Can Best Help a Dying Patient and His Family

1. Give helpful medical care and physical and emotional support. The patient should be assured that his pain and discomfort will be alleviated.

---

2. He should be honest with his patient and family about the seriousness of his diagnosis.
3. He should maintain some short-term hope while still being realistic.
4. He should not tell the patient when he is going to die, so that the patient gives up and waits for death.
5. He should try to show tenderness and interest by anticipating little things to make his patient more comfortable. He should make his patient feel that he is an individual rather than a health-care chart number.[2]

How to Minister to the Dying

You do not need to be a trained health-care professional to help someone who is terminally ill. You can be a family member, a friend, a hospice volunteer, or a fellow church member.

Ministering to a dying person can be much the same as ministering to a chronic situationer. Refer back to chapter 11 for those specifics.

Common fears of the dying: fear that death is the end; fear of losing consciousness, fear of loneliness as he or she is separated from those with life has been shared, fear of the unknown, fear of punishment based upon ideas of heaven and hell; fear of what may happen to those who depend on him or her; fear of failure.

Hopes for the dying: hope for relief from pain and fatigue; hope for blessings beyond; hope for finding loved ones who have gone before; hope for meeting God.

The dying person must be allowed to accept the diagnosis at his or her own pace. Most are willing to talk about the reality of the situation but after a few minutes change their minds. That is an indication they don't want to discuss it further.

It is natural for the dying person to wish to be with close friends and relatives. Their presence provides much comfort during this time. Their understanding and concern can reduce the loneliness of dying. Sometimes the dying person wants to speak privately with a family member or a friend. These intimacies provide a time in which the dying person can "put his affairs in order." Often funeral arrangements, matters of the will, and matters of both short- and long-term significance are discussed. After these matters are taken care of the dying person will feel a big relief and experience more peace about his upcoming death.

Isolation from loved ones is scary. In the Garden of Gethsemane, following the last supper, three times Jesus begged his disciples to stay with him. "My soul is overwhelmed with sorrow to the point of death. Stay here and keep watch with me" (Matthew 26:38). The loneliness and isolation prompted him to wake them three times—to give him the comfort of their presence, to fill the very human need of the presence of another in a time of great crisis. He tried to get some kind of support from his disciples, and all they did was sleep.

When a person is given a serious diagnosis, it forces him to look at himself and rearrange his priorities. "What the person *is* and *does* during the remainder of his life span is of major importance: that is what his life encompasses in feeling and understanding."[3] One man who had widespread abdominal cancer said, "Death is nothing. It is inevitable. Everyone has to die. What matters is *how* you live and die."[4] One dying person recorded his childhood memories in his last weeks of life, as a legacy for his children.

When a dying person realizes all the losses that have occurred in his life, plus the future losses he must face, he can become very depressed. Don't try to cheer him up or tell him to look on the brighter side of life. If he is allowed to express his sorrow, he will find a final acceptance easier. He will be grateful to those who can sit with him during this time. He will appreciate your listening, holding his hand, or hugging him.

The one emotion that usually persists through all the stages is hope. The dying person needs to maintain some hope in spite of a serious diagnosis. Perhaps there is a new drug or treatment that can be used. The first heart transplant patient must have felt that he was chosen to play a very special role in life. This hope enables the dying person to endure more painful tests and procedures.

If the doctor reassures the patient that he will do anything to keep him comfortable, the patient has the hope he needs and will not feel abandoned by the

medical profession. Some people want to travel or take up a hobby. He or she should try to fulfill desires if at all possible. The Make A Wish foundation was formed just so that dying children could have favorite wishes fulfilled.

Once it has been determined that no further treatments or procedures will reverse the dying process, medical treatment is no longer in order. The person has the right to decline any further treatments without friends and family inflicting guilt. Each dying person needs to make those decisions.

If the dying person wants to talk about the future, do not ignore his comments. Listening quietly can be a great service. Offer to stay with your friend while the family has time away. It's possible that she does not want to burden family members with all that she's feeling; a good friend nearby makes it possible for her to have the emotional release of sharing what's going on inside.

> *We have learned that for the patient, death itself is not the problem, but dying is feared because of the accompanying sense of hopelessness, helplessness, and isolation.—Elisabeth Kübler-Ross*

When a dying person is getting weaker, he can still remain as independent as possible. He should be getting up and going to bed, going to the bathroom, and getting dressed and undressed as long as he can. Have a chair close by that is easy to get in and out of. Eliminating the use of stairs provides more energy for other things. Create a place in which friends and relatives can visit with the dying person.

A hospice chaplain shares how to minister in tenderness. He says, "In the last moments and hours of life, people need guidance and support through the unknown and the mystery. Be there at the bedside with loving touches, gentle words and great tenderness. . . . Speak gently, clearly, simply. . . . Share your tears and the feelings that seem unacceptable. . . . Help in the physical care of your loved one. Bathe the feet. Massage the hands. Gently hold the head and smooth the hair. Lubricate the lips and mouth. Share memories—the playful, the inspirational, the ordinary. Humor and laughter are important."[5]

Sometimes the dying person needs quiet. Respect that and continue to be very near with your love.

It is important for the dying person to make final arrangements. This gives him the sense of his own worth and dignity to assume responsibility for preparing for his dying and death. These arrangements can pertain to finances, the funeral, and whatever else is on the agenda of the dying person.

It is often necessary for the dying person to separate himself from his family and loved ones. He needs to have permission from them to die at peace. The family needs to detach themselves and let go. This distancing phase is the most difficult, and family members should not view it as an insult.

The Family of the Dying

You cannot help the terminally ill person in a meaningful way if you do not include her family. Those in chronic situations need to deal with death and dying. It is not an easy or comfortable thing to discuss. Some people might view the whole idea as something that is quite morbid. Health personnel note that the families who have discussed these issues with the dying person seemed better equipped to cope with the death of their loved one. They seemed to have a better understanding of the person's feelings on this issue.

It is important that the terminal illness does not totally disrupt a household. The illness should allow for a gradual adjustment and change as to what kind of home it is going to be when the person is no longer around. Family members should not exclude all activities for the sake of being with the person. It is important that the dying person know that the family is able to function and carry on with their living without him.

Also families should refrain from laying guilt upon themselves: "If only I had sent him to a doctor earlier, maybe this wouldn't have happened." No one needs that guilt, and we have to remember that, ultimately, our lives are in God's hands.

When a terminal patient receives care at home, the patient and family need to decide about life-prolonging measures. They are under no obligation to call emergency services to resuscitate the dying person whose heart has stopped. However, families should remember that if they do call the paramedics who come with the ambulance, they are under standing orders to perform cardio-pulmonary resuscitation. Families of dying persons should consider in advance whether to call paramedics or not. All the caregivers—family members, doctor, home nurse, members of a hospice—should compile a list of directives that covers:

- what to do for pain or agitation
- what to do for breathing distress
- what to do when breathing stops
- when to call and when not to call the rescue squad

Ethical wills

You can pass on possessions through a traditional will. In the last few years living wills are becoming more common and these were discussed in chapter 12.

The *ethical will* is a Jewish tradition dating back to biblical times. Such a will may explain the reasons behind "why" the distribution of possessions is the way it is. Before her death, one mother called each family member into her bedroom and asked if there was a certain personal item that they would want as a reminder of her.

The main purpose of an ethical will is to pass on some of the lessons you've learned in life. A person writing this will also include Scripture passages that have been significant, along with hopes and dreams he or she has for the family. It is also a means of clearing up any unfinished business.

Rabbi Jack Reimer and Nathaniel Stampfer have written a book entitled *So That Your Values Live On—Ethical Wills and How to Prepare Them*. In many ways an ethical will should have the highest priority because it contains the religious values that have shaped your life. These have eternal value.

Hospice

At some point you may need hospice care. The hospice program originated near London in 1967 at St. Christopher's Hospice. The word *hospice* means "doors open to travelers on a journey from one life to the next." The hospice program provides supportive care for terminally ill patients and their families.

Hospice is care—not cure. Hospice providers are concerned about quality of life—not prolonging life. Hospice care stresses controlling the pain so the patient is comfortable physically but also spiritually and emotionally. "The pain that too often comes with terminal illness is an utter waste. It does not serve to warn or to instruct. It simply blots out, at one of the most important moments of our lives, all ability to perceive, to think sanely, or to be in any way master of the situation."[6]

> *You matter because you are you. You matter to the last moment of your life, and we will do all we can not only to help you die, peacefully, but also to live until you die.—Cicely Saunders*

Melissa Kelly, in her booklet "Using Hospice Care When A Loved One Is Dying," relates how she, her sisters, and parents tried to care for her eighty-eight-year-old grandmother. Before they found a hospice, they had little energy for anything but caring for the grandmother at home. They felt that as a loving family they should be able to cope with this situation. They turned to a hospice for help. The hospice team understood what a difficult time they were having.

The hospice setting may be a special unit in a hospital, a building in the community, or the home of the patient. Family members are urged to help with the patient's care as much as possible.

If you are interested in the hospice approach and would like to find out if there are hospice programs available in your area write to:

National Hospice Organization
1901 N. Moore St., Suite 901
Arlington, VA 22209
(703) 243-5900

Physical Symptoms of Death

Talking about symptoms of dying can seem morbid, but having some basic information helps us deal with death and avoid panic in situations where death is *not* occurring.

First of all, the dying person experiences gradual weakening of his body. He is very fatigued and often experiences colds and fevers that rapidly reduce his strength. The person may suffer weight loss and loss of appetite. He may experience nausea at the sight of food, vomiting after a meal, and constipation.

All this weakness can cause depression and misery. He may become fearful that he is becoming a burden to the family. The physician can help by prescribing an antidepressant which will decrease some of the lethargy he is experiencing.

> *Those who have the strength and love to sit with a dying person in the "silence that goes beyond words" will know that this moment is neither frightening nor painful, but a peaceful cessation of the functioning of the body.—Elisabeth Kübler-Ross*

Many times a dying person is conscious, although quite weak, immediately before death. The presence of the family at this time must be a comfort. When the dying person seems unconscious, the sense of hearing remains and should be considered.

Breathing, prior to death, may follow a cycle of shallow and then a deeper breath. This is called Cheyne-Stokes Respiration. Breathing may stop for about 5 to 30 seconds before the next cycle of shallow breathing begins. (Note: this breathing pattern can also occur in elderly people when they have taken sleeping pills.) Do not be alarmed if the person's breathing makes groaning or croaking sounds. It does not mean that he is in pain. When a dying person slips into a coma, the position of the neck and body produces the noise. This can be avoided by gently turning the person's shoulder or body.

A dying person can also develop a "death rattle." This happens because the unconscious person cannot cough up the secretions that build up in the back of the throat.

A pallor and stillness typically occur with death.

Within a few minutes of death the eyes become staring and the muscles of the face sag.

If the family is present at the moment of death, it is comforting for them to stay quietly at the bedside with their thoughts. Relatives often need a chance to touch, kiss, or just hold their loved one.

When no one is present at death, it is still a shock for the member of the family who first enters the room. It is helpful if that person tidies up the bedclothes and combs the person's hair before telling the rest of the family.

Procedures after Death

If the deceased indicated he wanted to donate any useful organs for transplants, these parts will be taken from the body at this time.

A death certificate will be issued and signed by a physician familiar with the deceased or the physician who was in attendance at the time of death. If the person died in a hospital, the certificate can be obtained from the business office along with any personal effects belonging to the deceased. In the event of an accidental or unexplained death, the certificate will be issued by the medical examiner's or coroner's office.

At this time the family must decide if they want an autopsy performed. An autopsy is required in the case of most accidents or if the deceased had not been seen by a physician within a specified time period. The autopsy can provide the family with specific information concerning the cause of death.

A clergy member should be called. Often he can give advice as to which funeral director is best. The funeral director then obtains permission to remove the body to the funeral home.

Someone must take charge of affairs and most families look to one or two family members to do this. It can be the eldest child of the deceased or a trusted friend.

The family lawyer should be appraised of the death and will be able to help in case the deceased has left any special instructions.

Ministering to the Grieving

When a friend or relative dies, our immediate reaction may be shock, sorrow, or disbelief. If the death was an unexpected one you too may react in shock. If death was expected, you may still feel uneasy about how to help the sorrowing.

Communicate in some way immediately upon hearing that death has occurred. Short visits to the home can be good. Phone calls let the bereaved know that you will help in any way. Praying together can give needed spiritual and physical strength. Pray for guidance for the family.

Encourage the immediate family members to make decisions regarding the funeral and burial. This helps them focus on the reality of what has happened. Many experts urge families to view the body of the deceased or have an open-coffin at the mortuary or the church.

Offer to call out-of-town relatives and friends. Help by volunteering to shuttle incoming relatives to and from the airport. Offer your home as a motel for visitors. Be there but do not take over the responsibilities of the family.

Encourage the grieving to talk about what has happened. Listen to them. Hug them. Sit beside them and cry with them. Avoid saying, "Don't cry. You'll be okay if you keep trusting the Lord. It happened for a purpose. God needed your loved one more than you do. I understand how you feel." Be willing to be silent.

Visit the mortuary. Signing your name in the guest book tells the family you cared enough to show respect for their loved one. Reading the guest book later on is a great comfort to the family. Attend the funeral or memorial service.

Don't be afraid to talk about the person who has died. It can be such a blessing to the family if you talk about experiences you had with the deceased. Even humorous anecdotes are welcome and needed.

Send flowers either to the home or mortuary. If the family requests no flowers, send a memorial in honor of the deceased. Often funeral expenses are great and if you can help financially, it is very much appreciated.

Help in any way during the busy times surrounding the death. Do be specific in your offers. Many churches have committees that organize meals for the bereaved. Encourage helpers to bring meals in disposable or marked containers. Offer to do errands, help with housework, etc. Offer to babysit if there are small children in the family.

As much as possible children should be included in the death and dying experience. Children can sense that something special is going on and it's good for them to be included.

Send a card. A sympathy card can say what you would want to but don't know how. Use expressions like, "It's hard to understand such things" or "My heart goes out to you." The bereaved can read these cards over and over and take comfort from them. Even if weeks have passed since the death occurred, write anyway. You could suggest meeting for lunch at a later date.

After the funeral, continue to communicate. Drop by for a short visit. Telephone to see how things are going. Often everyone goes their own ways and the bereaved are left to cope alone. Allow the bereaved to grieve. Listen to them go over the same memories again and again. Allow the cycle of emotions—tears, anger, fatigue, depression, and finally an adjustment of the loss. Everyone grieves differently.

> *But if grief is resolved, why do we still feel a sense of loss come anniversaries and holidays, and even when we least expect it? Why do we feel a lump in the throat, even six years after the loss? It is because healing does not mean forgetting, and because moving on with life does not mean that we don't take a part of our lost loved one with us.—Adolfo Quezada*

As time goes on, encourage the grieving to be involved in new activities. Suggest going to a Bible study together or to a support group.

The Funeral

There is no "right" way to bury someone you love, no perfect funeral plan. We would hope that everyone's funeral would assume some of the personality of the deceased. Your family should plan the funeral to honor the memory of him or her and at the same time give comfort to the family.

Often families are present at the time of death. Seeing and touching the dead body of your loved one is important to helping your family face your loss. In some religious traditions, relatives prepare the body. Some funeral directors will allow the family to help prepare the body for burial. Some people feel that having an open coffin and viewing the deceased's body makes death more real. When you see a lifeless corpse in a coffin, you know that all human relationships are ended with that person.

Many details must be attended to in a few short days: choosing a coffin, cemetery plot, when the family will be available to receive visitors at the mortuary or home, organizing the funeral service. All these decisions must be made in a few short days.

Many families ask that memorial gifts be made to the deceased's favorite charity. A flag may be draped over a veteran's coffin, or a favorite stuffed toy in the coffin of a child. I want my "empty" wheelchair parked next to my coffin to symbolize the fact that I won't need it anymore. "One family invited friends to contribute photos and drawings for a collage which now hangs in the living room as a last tribute to a lifetime."[7] Some families have a "memory table" on which are placed pictures or hobbies that are reminders of the deceased.

Some want their funeral services to be celebrations of resurrection instead of morbid services. Often memorial services are held a week or ten days after burial. Favorite hymns, music, comforting Scripture and poetry are part of these services. A time can be provided in which relatives and friends can share with the group what the deceased meant to them. Many Christians want their funerals to be a time in which the living are challenged with the gospel message.

> *I cannot honestly remember who was at the funeral home or the cemetery when Robbie died, but I have an overall recollection of being surrounded—almost cushioned—by people. Now, there are times when I go through the messages of condolence and the chapel visitors' book signed by those who attended the funeral, and I am still grateful for whatever time people gave us out of their lives. It was not easy for them, but it did an immeasurable amount of good for us.—Harriet Sarnoff Schiff*

It is biblical to grieve for our loved ones. The Bible does say that we should not "grieve like the rest of men, who have no hope" (1 Thessalonians 4:13). Christians have the hope that Christ will return and triumph over death.

Funerals are never the last word or the last event for those who believe in Jesus Christ. He said it himself: "he who believes has everlasting life" (John 6:47). Jesus is the Lord of life even though diseases and accidents destroy our physical bodies.

Helping Children Deal with Death

When a loved one is dying or death has occurred, the children are often the forgotten ones. Very few people feel comfortable talking to a child about death.

Our children were ages five, three, and one when my first porphyria attack happened. I came very close to death. While I was hospitalized our cat killed a bird and our children saw this. A few days after I came home from the hospital, a baby kitten died. Then one evening our three-year-old fell into an old well shaft filled with water. Tom found Luke clinging to the edge of the well and sputtering, "I thought I was going to die. I don't want to die." We didn't have a choice as to whether we wanted to talk to our children about death. We couldn't ignore it. They felt surrounded by death and illness.

Perhaps a young friend chases a ball into the street and is hit by a car. The child is rushed away in an ambulance and is never seen again.

A kindergarten child struggles with leukemia. Children see her on the playground wearing a hat because she's lost her hair. Then she dies.

Grandma has been struggling with poor health for years. When she dies, everyone is sad and quiet. They never see Grandma again.

Many times parents don't know what they think about death themselves, much less how to tell children about death. How much should they be told? Should they attend the funeral or mortuary? What if they see adults cry?

Up to the age of three a child is concerned mostly about separation. They cry when they are left in a nursery or at a babysitter. They are beginning to venture out into the world.

When a child is three–six years old, he may see a dead bird or squirrel, or have a pet that dies. This can provide opportunities to learn that death means not moving, not breathing, not seeing, and not making any sounds.

A child under the age of six cannot understand that death is irreversible and may expect the parent to bring a dead pet back to life. They see this in TV cartoons where the character is killed and bounces back to life again. The child may ask repeatedly: "Where did Grandma go? When is she coming back?"

After the age of eight or nine, children start to understand that death is final. They can have an adult understanding of death but they often personify death as a ghost or devil that comes to take people away. It helps if an adult can share a childhood experience about death and help them ease their fears.

No matter how mature a child is, it is difficult to understand that someone in the family is dying or has died. It is important for the children to know the family is united and to be involved in caring for the ill relative, if possible. They should be part of the team. They can sense that something dreadful is happening and adults are crying and worried. A "fear" fills the house and they may imagine something worse than the truth.

A child should simply be told that a loved one is dying. Then there should be time for the child to ask questions, and those questions need to be answered honestly. Keep explanations simple and brief. And children should not be shielded from the tears of adults; they need to know that adults are capable of expressing strong feelings—but they also need to see that life goes on.

It is not helpful to tell children, "Grandma went away on a long trip" or "she just went to sleep." They will learn not to trust an adult who answers in this way. They may become afraid to travel or to go to sleep.

Give a child the opportunity to participate in this event of death and dying. Children should not be forced but should be offered the opportunity to visit a dying person, attend a funeral or wake, witness a burial, or make a sympathy call with an adult. Simply explaining the proceedings can give them the necessary information they need. If a child does not want to see the body, the family must respect that decision and not force this on a child.

Each child processes grief in his own way. He may become aggressive or indifferent. Or he may seem grief-stricken or guilty. He may want to go out and play when grownups come to express sympathy. Adults should encourage the child to discuss his feelings, and an adult should be near to guide these discussions. It is normal for a child to have feelings of anger and loneliness.

There are no exact ways to help children through grief. Children have a way of surprising adults with some of the ideas and comments they have on death and dying. Honesty is necessary when you don't have answers to their questions. They need to be assured that you love them and will be close by.

Hospice groups offer classes for grieving children and their parents. Children learn, along with adults, that with time grief becomes less painful. These experiences can cement an adult-child relationship.

Encouragement along the Way

Words on Death and Dying

- "Don't treat me like a leper. Don't separate your-selves from me no matter how ugly I become in disposition or in appearance. Don't fail to see me because you won't know what to say or because you might cry, or for any other excuse you might discover to escape my presence. . . . When I die, my husband loses his wife, his lover, his confidante. My children lose their mother. Each friend loses me as a friend. But I lose all human relationships. . . . That's the meaning of being alone." —JoAnn Kelly Smith, *Free Fall*[8]

- "Will you turn me out if I can't get better?"—patient entering a London hospice in the 1960s

- "I don't want to die because I was made to live and life with all its relationships is so precious and valuable. But when the time comes my only concern will be the 'process of dying' and what that will involve. I don't fear death, only dying. Death is a friend to give me the ultimate victory that Jesus purchased for me, when all the struggles, vulnerabilities, and weaknesses of this life will be traded in for glory."

- "I am most certain that the problem in communication is much more with my colleagues and others than it is within myself. This is not to assess blame but to indicate the profundity with which an ill and dying person must take the burden of trying to communicate to others. And when this communication does not work, the dying person has the additional burden of helping the other person with his reactions. This is an unfair burden for me . . . yet if one is to stay in touch, it does become necessary for the dying person to take the initiative to assume responsibility in order to maintain the contact."— Archie Hanlan[8]

- "My dying is a fulfillment of God's promise for life eternally with Him—no more pain, no more tears—the glory of being in God's presence. The final stage of my life cycle."

Epilogue

> *Train yourself to be godly. For physical*
> *training is of some value, but godliness has*
> *value for all things, holding promise for both*
> *the present life and the life to come.*
> *—1 Timothy 4:7-8*

We have discussed and dealt with many issues—sometimes difficult ones. I feel as if I have given birth to this manuscript. Writing it has been a type of catharsis, bringing back positive and negative emotions. What lessons can be learned through our suffering?

We are waiting in a passage on our journey to heaven. We shouldn't fear tomorrow or live in the past. We never know who we will become and that's why life is called a journey. Suffering is guaranteed for anyone who takes on the task of living.

> *Life is a voyage that's homeward bound.*
> *—Herman Melville*

There are a few things we need to keep in mind during the journey.

God is in control and helps us in our pain, suffering, and dying. His faithfulness is our confidence in an uncertain future. We need to have a willingness to go without all the answers.

We learn that our loved ones are precious and we want to spend time with them. The only commodities that transfer from this life to the next are our relationships.

The experiences in our lives can help us mature so that we can live life more fully. Even how we die says a lot to others. One of the best things we can do for our brothers and sisters in Christ is to gain victory in our own trials.

When we have no way to turn, we realize that we need God's faithfulness and love. When we aren't able to trust, our sisters and brothers trust for us.

> *It is not what you do for Christ that counts; it is what you let him do through you.*—*Tom Carter*

A chronic situation gives many opportunities to show Christian concern and love for others. We need to ask ourselves, "Would I have done as much with my life if I had not had my chronic situation?"

The miracle of our existence on the earth has given our family a new awareness of God's love. The number of people who have prayed us through the last thirteen years extends to many people we don't even know. We'll meet these people in heaven and say thanks.

Being in a chronic situation causes us to ask some basic questions about life, such as, "What is happiness?" As children, we may have believed that a certain toy would make us happy. "If only I had a date to the prom, then I'd be happy." "If only—" Even as adults we look for happiness in big and expensive things and are miserable because we find that things don't make us happy.

Psychologists did a survey and found that happy people enjoy what they have rather than searching for what they don't have.

> *The great victories of life are oftenest won in a quiet way, and not with alarms and trumpets.*
> —*Benjamin N. Cardoza*

Being in a chronic situation causes us to reevaluate our priorities because we know that we do not have all the time in the world. Flare-ups and setbacks constantly remind us that we had better enjoy each day. From that experience chronic situationers often keep themselves focused. We notice the precious details of life and find pleasure in the "ordinary."

As we cope with our illness or disability, we can merely survive—or we can thrive. We thrive by accepting the situation and making it as good as possible, by getting the spiritual nourishment we need from God's Word and God's people, by putting into practice the faith lessons of love and service, by taking joy in gifts large and small, and, ultimately, by remembering that heaven awaits us.

Encouragement along the Way

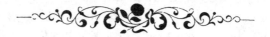

*S*ome Thoughts on Heaven

- "The way to Heaven is ascending; we must be content to travel uphill, though it be hard and tiresome, and contrary to the natural bias of our flesh."—Jonathan Edwards
- "If God were not willing to forgive sin, Heaven would be empty."—German Proverb
- "He who thinks most of heaven will do most for earth." —Anonymous
- "Do not let your hearts be troubled. Trust in God; trust also in me. In my Father's house are many rooms; if it were not so, I would have told you. I am going there to prepare a place for you. And if I go and prepare a place for you, I will come back and take you to be with me that you also may be where I am. You know the way to the place where I am going."—Jesus, in John 14:1-4
- "The gates of heaven are so easily found when we are little, and they are always standing open to let children wander in."—Sir James Matthew Barrie, *Sentimental Tommy* (Charles Scribner's Sons)
- "Things learned on earth, we shall practise in heaven." —Robert Browning
- "We talk about Heaven being so far away. It is within speaking distance to those who belong there."—Dwight L. Moody

- "Earth has no sorrow that Heaven cannot heal."—Sir Thomas Moore
- "God has two dwellings, one in heaven, and the other in a meek and thankful heart."—Izaak Walton
- "No eye has seen, no ear has heard, no mind has conceived what God has prepared for those who love him."—1 Corinthians 2:9

In light of what Jesus has done for us, we do not have to fear death. Nor should we long for it, because there is a purpose for our lives on earth. Having an anticipation for heaven is not being an escapist. The ultimate fulfillment that is talked about in the Scriptures we can find only in heaven.

Appendix A:

Living Will and Advance Directive

A Living Will and Durable Power of Attorney for Health Care
Plus Guide to Completion*

To my family, my friends, my doctors and all those concerned:

Directive made this _____day of _____, 19__.

I, _____ (name), being an adult of sound mind, willfully and voluntarily make this directive to be followed if I become incapable of participating in decisions regarding my medical treatment.

1. If at any time I should have an incurable or irreversible condition certified to be terminal by two medical doctors who have examined me, one of whom is my attending physician, or when use of life-sustaining treatment would only serve to artificially prolong the moment of my death, I direct that the expression of my intent be followed and that my dying not be prolonged. I further direct that I receive treatment necessary to keep me comfortable and to relieve pain.

*This living will and advance directive is © 1990 by the Hemlock Society and is used by permission. For a copy, send $3.50 check to:

The Hemlock Society
P.O. Box 11830
Eugene, OR 97440

INITIAL ONE:

___ I would like life-sustaining treatment, including artificial nutrition and hydration, to be withdrawn or withheld.[1]

___ I would like life-sustaining treatment withdrawn or withheld, but artificial nutrition and hydration continued.

Additional Instructions[2]: _____

_____

2. I appoint _____, residing at _____, as my agent, to make medical treatment decisions on my behalf, consistent with this directive.[3]

3. If I have been diagnosed as pregnant and that diagnosis is known to my physician, this directive shall not be effective during the course of my pregnancy.[4]

4. This directive shall have no force and effect after ____ years from the date of its execution, nor, if sooner, after revocation by me either orally or in writing.[5]

5. I understand the full importance of this directive and am emotionally and mentally competent to make this living will.

Signed _____

City, County and State of Residence _____

Caution: Check the numbered footnotes.
Some provisions may not apply to you.

WITNESSES TO LIVING WILL

The declarant is personally known to me and I believe her/him to be an adult and of sound mind.

I am not[6]:

1. Related to the declarant by blood or marriage;
2. Entitled to any portion of the declarant's estate either by will or codicil, or according to the laws of intestate succession;
3. Directly financially responsible for the declarant's medical care;
4. The declarant's doctor or an employee of that doctor;
5. An employee or patient in the hospital where the declarant is a patient.

_____   _____
Witness   Address

_____   _____
Witness   Address

NOTARIZATION[7]

State of _____)
)ss.
County of _____)

Subscribed and sworn to before me by _____,
Declarant and _____, witnesses, as the
voluntary act and deed of the declarant this _____ day of
_____, 19__.

My commission expires:

                            _____
                            Notary Public

GUIDE TO COMPLETION

1. Missouri and Wyoming statutes appear to mandate the provision of artificial nutrition and hydration. We recommend that you state your wishes, in any event.

2. Include any related expressions of your intent; for example, organ donation, that you wish to die at home, specific types of treatment you do not want, such as cardiopulmonary resuscitation (CPR) or antibiotics, etc.

3. 10 states and the District of Columbia have passed Durable Power of Attorney for Health Care statutes as of 1989; provisions in all states' general Power of Attorney statutes can be read to include health-care decisions. We recommend that you execute a Power of Attorney in addition to a Living Will, designating an individual to make health-care decisions in the event of your incapacity or disability. If you choose not to name an agent, draw a line through that part of the directive and initial it.

4. Many states have provisions in their Living Will statutes regarding pregnancy. If you do not desire this provision in your living will, draw a line through that part of the directive and initial it, keeping in mind that in the event of pregnancy, states with such a provision may enforce it.

5. A five year period is contained in California and North Dakota statutes only. If this does not apply to you and you wish your directive not to expire, draw a line through that part of the directive and initial it.

6. Because over half of the states with Living Will statutes contain all or some of these restrictions, we recommend that you choose witnesses who are not in any of these categories. If you are a resident of Georgia, a third witness is required when the directive is signed in the hospital. If you are in a nursing home, the following states require that one witness be a patient advocate or ombudsperson: California, Delaware, District of Columbia, North Dakota, and South Carolina.

7. Notarization, in addition to witnessing, is required in the following states: Hawaii, New Hampshire, North Carolina, Oklahoma, South Carolina and West Virginia. It is suggested by the statutes in Colorado and Tennessee. Alaska and Minnesota allow *either* signature by two witnesses *or* notarization.

ADVANCE DIRECTIVE INFORMATION

Name: _____   Social Security #: _____

Date of Birth: _____   Medical Record No.: _____

Please read the following statements:
Place your initials after *each* statement.

- I have been given written materials
  about my right to accept or refuse medical treatments and I have received a policy on Advance Directives.   _____
- I have been informed of my rights to execute Advance Directives.   _____
- I understand that I am not required to
  have an Advance Directive in order to receive medical treatment at this health
  care facility.   _____
- I understand that the terms of any Advance Directive that I have executed will
  be followed by the health care facility and
  my caregivers to the extent permitted by
  law.   _____

Please check one of the following statements:

☐ I have executed an Advance Directive and it meets
   my current wishes.

☐ I have not executed an Advance Directive.

Signed _____   Date _____

Witness _____   Date _____

261

Appendix B:
Additional Resources

The Resource Desk at your local public library can help you get associated with your health condition. For instance, if you have cancer, you could obtain the American Cancer Society's address from this resource.

Another way of finding materials pertaining to your chronic situation, is by checking the *Encyclopedia of Associations* at your public library.

American Hospital Guide to the Health Care Field is available in many libraries.

Be Sick Well by Jeff Kane, M.D. (Oakland, Calif.: New Harbinger Pub., 1991) provides a wealth of compassionate wisdom about "what to do" and "how to be" for people experiencing chronic illness.

Coming Home: A Guide to Dying at Home with Dignity by Deborah Duda (New York: Aurora Press, 1987).

Complete Directory for People with Disabilities (Grey House Publishers, n.d.).

Living with Sickness: A Struggle toward Meaning by Susan Saint Sing (Cincinatti: St. Anthony Messenger Press, 1987).

Long Term Health Care by Brickerner, Lechiah, Lipsman, Schare (New York: Basic Books, 1987).

Mainstay for the Well Spouse of the Chronically Ill by Maggie Strong (Boston: Little, Brown and Company, 1988).

A Reason to Live by Melody Beattie (Wheaton, Ill.: Tyndale Family Products, 1992).

Resource Directory for the Disabled by Richard Neil (Shrout New York: Contact Facts on File, 1991).

Super Joy by Paul Pearsall, Ph.D. (New York: Doubleday and Company, n.d.).

Yes You Can by Helynn Hoffa and Gary Morgan (New York: Pharos Books, 1990).

Magazines

A Positive Approach—A national Christian magazine for the physically challenged:
1600 Malone St.
Municipal Airport
Melville, NJ 08332

Accent on Living—Published quarterly and designed to meet the needs of the disabled:
P.O. Box 700
Bloomington, IL 61702

Organizations

American Cancer Society, Inc.
46 Fifth St. NE
Atlanta, GA 30308
(404) 816-7800
They publish the booklet "Questions and Answers about Pain Control."

National Chronic Pain Outreach Association
7979 Old Georgetown Rd., Suite 100
Bethesda, MD 20814-2429
(301) 652-4948
Laura S. Hitchwik, Ph.D. President
For $5 they will send you NCPOA's Starter Kit for support groups.

American Academy of Pain Management
3600 Sisk Rd.
Modesto, CA 95356
For $10 they will provide you with a list of all certified pain practitioners throughout the world.

Disability Rights Center
1346 Connecticut Ave. N.W.
Washington, D.C. 20036

American Pain Society
5700 Old Orchard Rd.
Skokie, IL 60077
(708) 966-5595

National Headache Foundation and
Diamond Headache Clinic
5252 North Western Ave.
Chicago, IL 60625
(312) 878-5558
Seymour Diamond, M.D., Executive Director

Arthritis Foundation
1314 Spring St. N.W.
Atlanta, GA 30309
(404) 872-7100
Don Riggin, President

Paralyzed Veterans of America
4350 East-West Highway, Suite 900
Bethesda, MD 20014
(301) 652-2135

Appendix C:
Questionnaires

These questionnaires were used to obtain information for the writing of this book. This was not a comprehensive survey; the information obtained was not used to generate statistics, but to gather honest responses from people in situations of chronic illness. Most of the respondents were from the Christian Reformed Church, and the questionnaires were handled through the church's Disability Concerns Office.

Questionnaire for Adults in Chronic Situations

1. Briefly describe your long-term chronic situation.

2. What do you fear the most about being ill or disabled—loss of money, time, activity, responsibilities?

3. During a setback, flare-up, or time of discouragement, what helps you the most? What are the steps you use to regain control of your condition?

4. During a flare-up, what is the best way that friends or family can help you?

5. Are you part of a support group? If you are, tell what ways this group has been helpful.

Questionnaire for Support
Person/Caregiver/Spouse/Other Family

1. What is your relationship to the person in your chronic or long-term situation?

2. What have you learned as a caregiver?

3. What helps you the most when you are tired and down about your chronic caregiving? Do you talk to a friend/take part in a support group/take time out alone?

4. Do you have any particular Scripture or prayers that help you the most? If any, please tell how they help you.

5. Any other comments are welcome.

Notes

Chapter 1

1. Sefra Kobrin Pitzele, *We Are Not Alone: Learning to Live with Chronic Illness* (New York: Workman Publishing, 1986), p. 12.

2. Gilda Radner, *It's Always Something* (New York: Simon and Schuster, 1989), p. 21.

Chapter 2

1. Michael Castleman, "Are You a Medical Mystery?", *The Reader's Digest* (February 1991), pp. 185-192.

2. Donald S. Pierce, and Vernon H. Nickel, *Total Care of Spinal Cord Injuries* (Boston: Little, Brown and Company, 1977), p. 52.

3. Robert Chernin Cantor, *And a Time to Live* (New York: Harper Colophon Books, 1978), p. 124.

4. Dr. Lewis B. Smedes, *A Pretty Good Person* (San Francisco: Harper and Row, 1990), p. 6.

5. Stanley C. Baldwin, *Bruised But Not Broken* (Portland, Oreg.: Multnomah Press, 1985), p. 36.

6. Annie Johnson Flint, *Hymns for the Family of God* (Nashville: Paragon Associates, 1976), p. 112.

Chapter 3

1. Betty Rollin, *First You Cry* (New York: Harper and Row, 1976), p. 240.

2. Claudia Black, *Double Duty* (New York: Ballantine Books, 1990), p. 480.

3. Bernice Wallin, *I Beat Cancer* (Chicago: Contemporary Books, 1978), p. 114.

4. Howard Vanderwell, *Proven Promises* (Hudsonville, Mich.: HDVW Press, 1990), p. 21.

5. Robert O. Beatty, *Still a Lot of Living: Coping with Cancer* (New York: Macmillan, 1978), n.p.

6. Richard H. Blum, *Doctors, Hospitals and Medical Care* (New York: Macmillan, 1964), p. 271.

7. Robert Chernin Cantor, *And a Time to Live* (New York: Harper Colophon Books, 1978), p. 13.

Chapter 4

1. Isadore Rosenfeld, M.D., *Second Opinion* (New York: The Linden Press/Simon and Schuster, 1981), p. 39.

2. David R. Stutz, M.D., and Bernard Feder, and the editors of *Consumer Reports Books, The Savvy Patient* (Mount Vernon, N.Y.: Consumers Unions, 1990), p. 1.

3. Richard H. Blum, *Doctors, Hospitals and Medical Care* (New York: Macmillan, 1964), p. 35.

4. Larrian Gillespie, M.D., *You Don't Have to Live with Cystitis* (New York: Rawson Associates, 1986), p. 4.

5. *Doctors, Hospitals and Medical Care,* p. 108.

6. *The Savvy Patient*, p. 78.

7. Jane Patterson, M.D., and Lynda Maclaras, *Woman Doctor* (New York: Avon Books, The Hearst Corp., 1983), p. 15.

8. Ibid., p. 31.

9. Norman Cousins, *Head First* (New York: E.P. Dutton, 1989), p. 117.

10. Mark Flapan, "Living with a Rare Disorder—What Do You Want from Your Dr.?" NORD (New Fairfield, Conn.: Spring 1990), p. 11.

11. Lanie Jones, "Learning Bedside Manners," *Los Angeles Times* (October 1, 1991).

12. Howard Markel, "Remembering Debby," *Good Housekeeping* (October 1991).

13. *The Savvy Patient*, p. 93.

14. *Second Opinion,* p. 373.

Chapter 5

1. Marlene Cimons, "Everett Koop," *Los Angeles Times* (February 23, 1992), p. M3.

2. Kenneth Lewis, "The Professional Nurse: Regardfully Necessary," *A Positive Approach* (Spring, 1991), p. 54.

3. Lillian Scholtis Brunner and Doris Smith Suddarth, *Textbook of Medical-Surgical Nursing* (Philadelphia: J.B. Lippincott, 1984), pp. 188-189.

4. John Ankerberg and John Weldon, *Can You Trust Your Doctor?* (Brentwood, Tenn.: Wolgemuth and Hyatt, 1991), p. 20.

5. Kenneth Anderson, *Orphan Drugs* (New York: The Linden Press/ Simon and Schuster, 1983), p. 123.

Chapter 6

1. Richard M. Linchitz, M.D., *Life without Pain* (New York: Addison-Wesley Publications, 1987), p. 9.

2. Ken Dachman and John Lyons, *You Can Relieve Pain* (New York: Harper and Row, 1990), p. 7.

3. Ibid., p. 19.

4. Edward J. Beattie Jr., with Stuart D. Cowan, *Toward the Conquest of Cancer* (New York: Crown Publishers, 1980).

5. Susan C. Pescor and Christine A. Nelson, M.D., *Where Does It Hurt?* (New York: Facts on File, 1983), p. 283.

6. Portland Pain Center staff, *A Guide to the Portland Pain Center* (Portland, Oreg., 1983), p. 2.

7. *Life without Pain*, p. 39.

8. *You Can Relieve Pain,* p. 39.

9. Ruth Pecor, "How to Live with Chronic Pain," *Handicap News* (April 1988), p. 6.

10. Anne Morrow Lindbergh, *Hour of Gold, Hour of Lead* (New York: Harcourt, Brace and Jovanovich, 1973), p. 252.

11. *Toward the Conquest of Cancer,* p. 186.

12. Anne C. Roark, "The Search for Relief of Pain," *Los Angeles Times* (September 22, 1991), p. A33.

13. Ibid.

14. *Toward the Conquest of Cancer,* p. 187.

15. "The Search for Relief of Pain," p. A33.

16. Stanley L. Englebardt, "Why Must They Suffer?" *Reader's Digest* (November 1990), p. 22.

17. "Poll Results—What Readers Say about Pain," *Accent on Living* (Summer 1991), p. 82.

18. Dorothy Snell, *Sent Home to Die* (Boise, Idaho: Pacific Press, 1987), p. 22.

19. JoAnn Kelley Smith, *Free Fall* (Valley Forge, Penn.: Judson Press, 1975), p. 94.

20. Tim Hansel, *Ya Gotta Keep Dancin'* (Elgin, Ill.: David C. Cook, 1985), p. 122.

21. Ibid., p. 123.

Chapter 7

1. Lucille Kulper, "Journey from Desolation," *Pine Rest Today* (Grand Rapids: Community Relations Department of Pine Rest Christian Hospital, Fall 1991), p. 3.

2. Sharon and David Sneed, "Why Am I So Depressed?" *Today's Christian Woman* (January/February 1991), p. 159.

3. "Journey from Desolation," p. 3.

4. Vera M. Robinson, *Humor and the Health Professions* (Thorofare, N.J.: Charles B. Slack, 1977), p. 134.

Chapter 8

1. Judi Johnson and Linda Klein, *I Can Cope* (Minneapolis: DCI Publishing, 1988), p. 148.

2. Dan Warrick, *How to Handle Stress* (Colorado Springs: NavPress, 1989), p. 5.

3. Helynn Hoffa and Gary Morgan, *Yes You Can: A Helpbook for the Physically Disabled* (New York: Pharos Books, 1990), p. 182.

4. Donald S. Pierce, M.D., and Vernon H. Nickel, M.D., *Total Care of Spinal Cord Injuries* (Boston: Little, Brown and Company, 1977), p. 304.

Chapter 9

1. Donald S. Pierce, M.D., and Vernon H. Nickel, M.D., *Total Care of Spinal Cord Injuries* (Boston: Little, Brown and Company, 1977), p. 304.

2. Georgia Photopulos and Bud Photopulos, *Of Tears and Triumphs* (New York: Congdon and Weed, 1988), p. 74.

3. Ibid., p. 75.

4. Iris Sneider, *Patient Power* (White Hall, Va.: Betterway Pub., 1986), p. 89.

5. Donald S. Pierce, M.D., and Vernon H. Nickel, M.D., *Total Care of Spinal Cord Injuries* (Boston: Little, Brown and Company, 1977), p. 305.

6. Betsy Burnham, *When Your Friend Is Dying* (Old Tappan, N.J.: Chosen Books, Fleming H. Revell, 1978), p. 76.

7. Sefra Kobrin Pitzele, *We Are Not Alone: Learning to Live with Chronic Illness* (New York: Workman Publishing, 1986), p. 64.

Chapter 10

1. Jane Royse, "Perspectives on Caregiving," *Advantage Magazine,* p. 9.

2. Georgia Photopulos and Bud Photopulos, *Of Tears and Triumphs* (New York: Congdon and Weed, 1988), p. xi.

3. Betsy Burnham, *When Your Friend Is Dying* (Old Tappan, N.J.: Chosen Books, Fleming H. Revell, 1978), p. 78.

4. *Of Tears and Triumphs,* p. 142.

5. Ann Landers, "Nursing Home Tips," *Daily Bulletin* (October 1991), p. B4.

6. Joni Eareckson Tada, *Secret Strength* (Portland, Oreg.: Multnomah Press, 1988), p. 56.

Chapter 11

1. Ann Landers, *Daily Bulletin* (January 18, 1992).

2. Sefra Kobrin Pitzele, *We Are Not Alone: Learning to Live with Chronic Illness* (New York: Workman Publishing, 1986), p. 59.

3. Roberta Lozes, "This Letter Was Our Call for Help," *Accent on Living* (Summer 1991).

4. Bert Zwiers, "Background" (March 1992).

5. Barbara Johnson, *Stick a Geranium in Your Hat and Be Happy* (Dallas, Tex.: Word, 1990), p. 54.

6. Ken Czillinger, "When Someone You Love Is Suffering," *Care Notes* (St. Meinrad, In.: Abbey Press, 1989), p. 1.

7. Jim R. Kok, "Ninety Percent of Helping Is Just Showing Up," *The Banner* (April 15, 1991).

8. Carol Luebering, "Looking for a Hug," *Care Notes* (St. Meinrad, In.: Abbey Press, 1988), p. 2.

9. *Stick a Geranium in Your Hat and Be Happy,* p. 28.

10. Jim R. Kok, "Healing the Whole Person," *The Banner* (December 14, 1987), p. 9.

11. Joni Eareckson Tada with Bev Singleton, *Friendship Unlimited* (Wheaton, Ill: Harold Shaw Publishers, 1987), p. 75.

12. Virginia Schneider, "Following in Stephen's Footsteps," *Guideposts* (May 1991), p. 21.

Chapter 12

1. Arnold A. Hutschnecker, *The Will to Live* (New York: Simon and Schuster, 1986), p. 19.

2. David R. Stutz, M.D., and Bernard Feder, and the editors of *Consumer Reports Books. The Savvy Patient* (Mount Vernon, N.Y.: Consumers Union, 1990), p. 217.

3. Irving S. Wright, "Who Should Make the Decisions?" in *The Moment of Death,* edited by Arthur Winter (Springfield, Ill.: Thomas, 1969).

4. Kenneth E. Schemmer, *Between Life and Death* (Wheaton, Ill.: Victor Books, 1988), p. 58.

5. Ibid., p. 41.

6. Ibid., pp. 38-39.

7. Janet Kaye, "The Long Goodbye," *Los Angeles Times* (July 14, 1991), p. 16.

8. Ibid.

9. "The Living Will," *Accent On Living* (Spring 1991), p. 51.

10. Ibid., p. 53.

11. *Between Life and Death,* p. 18.

12. Andrew C. Jubsch, "Zero Options," *Parents of Teenagers* (October/November 1991), p. 1.

13. Audrey T. Hingly, "I Found No Room for Miracles," *The Christian Reader* (January/February 1992), p. 60.

14. Russell Chandler, "Religion Confronts Euthanasia," *Los Angeles Times* (October 1991).

15. Ibid.

16. Ibid.

17. Ibid.

18. Ibid.

Chapter 13

1. JoAnn Kelly Smith, *Free Fall* (Valley Forge, Penn.: Judson Press, 1975), p. 100.

2. Richard H. Blum, *Doctors, Hospitals and Medical Care* (New York: Macmillan, 1964), p. 140.

3. Lawrence Le Shan, *You Can Fight for Your Life* (New York: M. Evans and Company, 1977), p. 98.

4. Ibid.

5. Roy H. Anderson, "Hospice Chaplain Shares How to Minister in Tenderness," *Good News, Etc.* (August 1991), p. 2.

6. Sandol Stoddard, *The Hospice Movement* (Briarcliff Manor, N.Y.: Stein and Day Publishers, 1978), p. 46.

7. Carol Luebering, "Planning the Funeral of Someone You Love," (St. Meinrad, Ind.: Abbey Press, 1988), p. 5.

8. *Free Fall,* n.p.

9. Archie Hanlan, *Autobiography of Dying* (Garden City, N.Y.: Doubleday, 1979), p. 31.

Bibliography

Anderson, Kenneth. *Orphan Drugs*. New York: The Linden Press/Simon and Schuster, 1983.

Ankerberg, John, and John Weldon. *Can You Trust Your Doctor?* Brentwood, Tenn.: Wolgemuth and Hyatt, 1991.

Baldwin, Stanley C. *Bruised But Not Broken*. Portland, Oreg.: Multnomah Press, 1985.

Beattie, Edward J., Jr. with Stuart D. Cowan. *Toward the Conquest of Cancer*. New York: Crwon Publishers, 1980.

Beatty, Robert O. *Still a Lot of Living: Coping with Cancer*. New York: Macmillan, 1978.

Black, Claudia. *Double Duty*. New York: Ballantine Books, 1990.

Blum, Richard H. *Doctors, Hospitals and Medical Care*. New York: Macmillan, 1964.

Bogin, Meg. *The Path to Pain Control*. Boston: Houghton Mifflin, 1982.

Brunner, Lillion Scholtis, and Doris Smith Suddareth. *Textbook of Medical-Surgical Nursing*. Philadelphia: J.B. Lippincott, 1984.

Burnham, Betsy. *When Your Friend Is Dying*. Old Tappan, N.J.: Chosen Books, Fleming H. Revell, 1978.

Cantor, Robert Chernin. *And a Time to Live*. New York: Harper Colophon Books, 1978.

Cousins, Norman. *Head First*. New York: E.P. Dutton, 1989.

Dachman, Ken, and John Lyons. *You Can Relieve Pain*. New York: Harper and Row, 1990.

Flint, Annie Johnson. *Hymns for the Family of God*. Nashville: Paragon Associates, 1976.

Flynn, Eileen P. *Hard Decisions*. Kansas City, Mo.: Sheen and Ward, 1990.

Fresne, Florine Du. *Home Care: An Alternative to the Nursing Home*. Elgin, Ill.: The Brother Press, 1983.

Gillespie, Larrian, M.D. *You Don't Have to Live with Cystitis.* New York: Rawson Associates, 1986.

Hanlan, Archie. *Autobiography of Dying.* Garden City, N.Y.: Doubleday, 1979.

Hansel, Tim. *Ya Gotta Keep Dancin'.* Elgin, Ill.: David C. Cook, 1985.

Hill, Margaret. *Coping with Family Expectations.* New York: The Rosen Publishing Group, Inc., 1990.

Hultschnecker, Arnold A. *The Will to Live.* New York: Simon and Schuster, 1986.

Johnson, Barbara. *Stick a Geranium in Your Hat and Be Happy.* Dallas, Tex.: Word, 1990.

Johnson, Judi and Linda Klein. *I Can Cope.* Minneapolis: DCI Publishing, 1988.

Kübler-Ross, Elisabeth. *On Death and Dying.* New York: Collier Books/Macmillan, 1969.

Landorf, Joyce. *The High Cost of Growing.* Nashville: Thomas Nelson, 1978.

Le Shan, Lawrence. *You Can Fight for Your Life.* New York: M. Evans and Company, 1977.

LeMaistre, JoAnn. *Beyond Rage: The Emotional Impact of Chronic Physical Illness.* Oak Park, Ill.: Alpine Guild, 1988.

Linchitz, Richard M., M.D. *Life without Pain.* New York: Addison-Wesley Publications, 1987.

Lindbergh, Anne Morrow. *Hour of Gold, Hour of Lead.* New York: Harcourt, Brace and Jovanovich, 1973.

Patterson, Jane, M.D., and Lynda Maclaras. *Woman Doctor.* New York: Avon Books, The Hearst Corporation, 1983.

Pescor, Susan C., and Christine A. Nelson, M.D. *Where Does It Hurt?* New York: Facts on File, 1983.

Photopulos, Georgia, and Bud Photopulos. *Of Tears and Triumphs.* New York: Congdon and Weed, 1988.

Pierce, Donald S., M.D., and Vernon H. Nickel, M.D. *Total Care of Spinal Cord Injuries.* Boston: Little, Brown and Company, 1977.

Pitzele, Sefra Kobrin. *We Are Not Alone: Learning to Live with Chronic Illness.* New York: Workman Publishing, 1986.

Portland Pain Center, staff. *A Guide to the Portland Pain Center.* Portland, Oreg.: Staff published, 1983.

Radner, Gilda. *It's Always Something.* New York: Simon and Schuster, 1989.

Robinson, Vera M. *Humor and the Health Professions*. Thorofare, N.J.: Charles B. Slack, 1977.

Rollin, Betty. *First You Cry*. New York: Harper and Row, 1976.

Rosenfeld, Isadore, M.D. *Second Opinion*. New York: The Linden Press/ Simon and Schuster, 1981.

Ryan, Dale, and Juanita Ryan. *Recovering from Loss*. Downers Grove, Ill.: InterVarsity Press, 1990.

Schemmer, Kenneth E. *Between Life and Death*. Wheaton, Ill.: Victor Books, 1988.

Smedes, Lewis B. *A Pretty Good Person*. San Francisco: Harper and Row, 1990.

Smith, JoAnn Kelley. *Free Fall*. Valley Forge, Penn.: Judson Press, 1975.

Sneider, Iris., A.C.S.W. *Patient Power*. White Hall, Va.: Betterway Pub., 1986.

Snell, Dorothy. *Sent Home to Die*. Boise, Idaho: Pacific Press, 1987.

Stewart, Clifford T., Ph.D. *Cancer*. Wallingford, Penn.: Hampton Court Press, 1988.

Stoddard, Sandol. *The Hospice Movement*. Briarcliff Manor, N.Y.: Stein and Day Publishers, 1978.

Stutz, David R., M.D., and Bernard Feder, and the editors of *Consumer Reports Books*. *The Savvy Patient*. Mount Vernon, N.Y.: Consumers Union, 1990.

Tada, Joni Eareckson, with Bev Singleton. *Friendship Unlimited*. Wheaton, Ill.: Harold Shaw Publishers, 1987.

Tada, Joni Eareckson. *Secret Strength*. Portland, Oreg.: Multnomah Press, 1988.

Vanderwell, Howard. *Proven Promises*. Hudsonville, Mich.: HDVW Press, 1990.

Wallin, Bernice. *I Beat Cancer*. Chicago: Contemporary Books, 1978.

Warrick, Dan. *How to Handle Stress*. Colorado Springs: NavPress, 1989.

Wheeler, Eugene G., and Joyce Dace-Lombard. *Living Creatively with Chronic Illness: Developing Skills for Transcending the Loss, Pain and Frustration*. Ventura, Calif.: Pathfinder, 1989.